Sociology
for
NURSES

Second Edition

Sociology for NURSES

Second Edition

GN Prabhakara
Principal and Professor of PSM
SDM College of Medical Sciences and Hospital
Dharwad, Karnataka

PEEPEE
PUBLISHERS AND DISTRIBUTORS (P) LTD.

Sociology for Nurses

Published by
Pawaninder P. Vij
Peepee Publishers and Distributors (P) Ltd.
7/31, First Floor, Ansari Road, Daryaganj, Post Box-7243
New Delhi-110002 (India)

Ph: 65195868, 23246245, 9811156083

e-mail: peepee160@yahoo.co.in

e-mail: peepee160@rediffmail.com

e-mail: peepee160@gmail.com
www.peepeepub.com

First Edition: 2004,2005,2007
Second Edition: 2009

ISBN: 81-8445-067-2

Printed at
Lordson, C-5/19, Rana Pratap Bagh, Delhi-110 007

Preface to the Second Edition

I am happy over latest edition after earlier edition and reprint of "**SOCIOLOGY FOR NURSES**" by Peepee Publishers and Distributors (P) Ltd., New Delhi.

Author's experience came into action when Mr. Pawaninder P Vij offered to score the text of "SOCIOLOGY FOR NURSES" which has given good response from teachers and the taught.

Syllabus as per Nursing Council of India is covered for the text. One chapter on social Trends and Social Issues is added. Society Sociology, Wealth Index, Human Poverty Index, Hospital Sociology, Population Sociology, Socio-demographic Impact, History of Sociology, Rural Classification, Trans-cultural Society, Group Dynamics, Industrialisation, Classification of Social Problems and Medical Social Worker, Community Development Programme including voluntary health agencies are added.

This updated and revised edition will meet the requirements of nursing profession. My appreciation to Mr. Pawaninder P Vij for the atmost care in the publication of the text.

Dr. GN Prabhakara
Dharwad, Karnataka
April 2009

Preface to the First Edition

Nursing profession commands higher scale of understanding, sympathy, advice, counselling and nursing care of the sick and injured. This involves the study of interaction of social phenomenon in and around us.

This was felt and conveyed in teaching and training of nurses at different levels. But to put forth the experience came to action when Mr Pawaninder P Vij offered to score the text **of Sociology for Nurses** based on the requirement of the teacher and taught. Hence the birth of the text is the credit and the credit goes to Mr Pawaninder P Vij.

I hope to see the *unmet need* **met with nursing profession in their endeavour.**

GN Prabhakara

Acknowledgements

Initiation, motivation, guidance, corrections, proof reading, specific appropriations and thorough help of my life partner Mrs.Malathi Prabhakara Ex Scientist, Technology Transfer, Industrial Development and Consultancy Services, CFTRI, CSIR, Mysore is highly acknowledged.

Source of inspiration of my son Dr. Bharat M P post graduate cum tutor in Radiodiagnois and Imaging at SDMCMS & H Dharwad is affectionately acknowledged.

Screening, advice and providing reference material by the subject expert, Sociologist Dr.Soumya Kumar Professor of Sociology, Maharani's College, Mysore is affectionately acknowledged.

I acknowledge the respect and regards bestowed upon me by nursing students and nursing professionals who inspired me to bring out my experience in the present form.

All the more with high appreciation the efforts of M/s. Peepee Publishers and Distributors (P) Ltd., New Delhi in giving a good commendable shape to my modest work are acknowledged with heartfelt thanks.

GN Prabhakara

CONTENTS

1

Introduction

One of the basic characteristics of a man is craving for sympathy, which attracts attention in normal life. However in illness he attracts a fundamental need *'the nursing'*.

Human being has many instincts, which made him to get transformed to physical change, mental change, physiological change and cultural change to rule over other living beings. He has the art of adding experience. This helped him to shape a better tomorrow. He developed social standards, which guided him to achieve progress, prosperity and health.

SOCIOLOGY

Sociology in contemporary usage has two meanings. One is broad with expression of the humanitarian tradition in nursing and public frequently read into it any interpretation consistent with their experience and interests. This defines the humane care of patients, prevention of disease, health education, nutrition education, counselling, the work of local health authorities, finance of nursing services and indeed concerned with health and welfare. The other is restricted sense in which we shall be using sociology with a body of knowledge and methods of obtaining that knowledge to nursing profession. In a nutshell, it studies the nursing need of the society and the human epidemiology.

The word SOCIOLOGY is derived from *socios* meaning *society* and *logos* meaning *study.*

Sociology along with psychology, psychiatry and anthropology determine and influence human behavior and thereby his interaction with the society is determined.

Let us take an illustration from nursing care;

Mrs. Pooja aged 52 years admitted for hysterectomy. She is admitted in Gynaec ward bed number 9. Duty nurse, ward nurse, head nurse and matron all give instructions like·

- Get biopsy report of bed number 9 DUB case
- Do not give food at night since the case is selected for morning surgery
- Which is the native place of DUB case.

Thus, all along attending surgical and general nursing profession never call Pooja by her name. Addressing her by name can bring a good nurse patient relationship. Pooja wanted to know how long the surgery takes place and what is done in operation for DUB? When attending nurse remains silent and non-communicative with patient, all patient questions remains unanswered. Here conducting herself by the attending nurse is utmost important in her professional duties.

Sociology provides an insight into the understanding of many events and activities that seem to concern our society, our family and our organisation. One has to think away from usual routines for proper understanding of sociology in nursing profession. To illustrate, a sister greets you in the ward "good morning". It has a symbolic value for your social activity. It provides occasion for your social interaction in human society. It is an accepted norm and not misbehavior. Moreover, if you are greeted you have commanded respect and regards in your position and you have life-style choice to greet her by any one of the following reciprocations;

- Bowing your head
- Raising your right hand to give a partial solute
- Raising your left hand to say "hoi"
- Namaste by both palm together

Sociology in nursing profession has an area of interest for the study of health, disease, health behavior and social medical interactions. We have many social illness (diseases) like:

- Tuberculosis
- Leprosy
- Sexually transmitted diseases
- AIDS.

Similarly nursing profession has an obligation to see that diet, therapy, counselling, assistance, defence and security apart from welfare through social obligations which we control in terms of:

- Social diet
- Social therapy
- Social counselling
- Social assistance
- Social defence
- Social security.

Society depends upon the quality of the individuals it produces. These individuals cannot work if they are over organised, if they are over legalised and if their urge to achieve greatness are suppressed; then we are sure that civilisation collapses. Early societies recognised human male to put their efforts to defend and care for children as biological father and protect their wives. The process of nuclear families must have started about 10000 years ago. Primitive societies developed codes and norms to preserve their families from which humanity was developed. Thus ancient codes or commandments are the root for the concept of justice.

Overall physical and mental development of children is possible by the fact that their biological father and mother in a family environment raise them. Patriarchal societies built on families thrived in terms of living standards and material wealth. A basic survival was seen in such families. Matriarchal societies have shown a tendency to regress. Patriarchal marriage identified the evolution of society. This has been there prior to the development of birth control and DNA testing.

Though civilisation ultimately rests on family, there is a perceptual change in the attitude of women and many women find marriage confining. Child rearing is no longer a lifetime occupation. Women tend to bear children much later in life. Human society has tried many permutations to find a better way of raising children. Time tested style of rising children in consonance with the then social norms has given way to shaping children to be more independent and aggressive. In this bargain, the existing societal norms as well as government regulation no longer finds its utility for the changing characteristics of the society. In history of man we have seen that if a country tries to create a political solution to human problems has ended up with gulags and concentration camps. In human societies there is hatredness of those who are different from a group.

Tolerance of religion, race, political persuasion, and tribal allegiances is a requisite in the overall advancement of human societies. Primitive societies have seen the punishment like Greek Hoplites, ostracism and shunning for homosexuality. Now homosexuality is being slowly being accepted as a part of social system and no longer being considered as social evil. It is now considered as a human condition comparable to skin colour or where they live. They are not treated as sub humans.

Perhaps what we need to examine is the evolution of a social system where all people with many beliefs and persuasions can form their own communities without persecution while enjoying the benefits and protections of a uniform rule of law. We can infer that a uniform social order means is to envision a disaster for human rights and progress.

Experimentation in societies is risky and sometimes even more detrimental to the society. Nazi Germany and the Soviet Union tried just that in mid twentieth century with tens of millions killed as an end result! Lenin when came to power in the Soviet Union after Soviet revolution, passed what amounts to our no-fault divorce statutes. This along with communist encouragement of sexual immorality during marriage, approval of abortion, and forcing women out of the house into the workforce accomplished its purpose of destroying the Russian social system viz., the family.

By the late 1800s evolutionary concepts were exercising a powerful influence throughout Western Civilisation. The utter brutality of evolutionary 'tooth and fang' teachings ravaged society on many levels. 'Survival of the fittest' became the hallmark of dictators, fanatics and social innovators.

Four stages of society's evolution:

Society has developed through overlapping stages of physical, vital, mental and spiritual stages. Physical realities like survival, life of fear and threat, need for complete deference to authority is known entities. Society has vital needs like desire to expand and trade. The mental stage is expressed through peace, freedom, democracy, the fulfilment and empowerment of the individual. The spiritual stage has multi sided awareness of truth that allow spiritual force for ultimate flowering and transformation of life.

Physical stage of evolution of society:

In Stone Age, man focused all his activities on his very survival and existence. All other things were secondary. Insecurity was an atmosphere in that age. There were threats from nature, from tribes and from other collectives. The social awareness was limited.

Vital stage of evolution of society:

This started with better cohesion and unity in collectives. Man mastered the basic productive operations of life, gained control of physical forces around him. This was the beginning of trade with other tribes and more interaction with others. Man got more exposure to outside world from his travel from place to place. Expansion of vitality in the vital stage brought forth change in man's attitude towards life, showed more interest in material life and thus became prosperous and enjoyed life.

Mental stage of evolution of society:

During this stage of evolution, Knowledge was gained through training and education. This stage brought in vast development in science, communication and technology of recent years. We could see freedom, initiative and self-determinism in man. The awareness and concern for the plight of others, the demand of the individual to be involved in the decisions of the collective, and the emerging political and social freedom are some of the indicators of the mental stage of social evolution.

Spiritual stage of evolution of society:

Man while emerging through mental stage perceived that even the power of mind could not be the ultimate salvation for humanity. He felt faculties of mind were limited. The quest for greater truths, greater insights, spiritual knowledge and vision was seen. Man felt individual will, collective will and Divine will all are bound together. Every body started opening themselves to a greater spiritual power to effect life called divine life on earth transforming them to a higher physical vital and physical existence to experience the spirit in action in life just as *Sri Aurobindo* envisioned his state beyond the mental stage, is the main essence of spiritual stage of evolution of society.

NURSE

The word nurse has come from the word nourishing, which means tending and helping all who need it, especially the sick. Her adequate service depends upon her understanding the mind and body of other individual in her skills used in nursing profession.

Nursing is the key component of health care in all socio economic setting. It ranges from carrying out high technology investigations like Aortogram to low technology first contact care like ORS preparation.

The nursing care is influenced by social context in which the activity is going to take place.

There is a force-field in nursing care and nursing practice, which either hinder or help to cater nursing care in the community.

Sociology in nursing aims at **Health For All**, a set out preamble of constitution of W.H.O. which gives positive health demarcating the line of action by nurse to serve both well and ill in the community, right to nursing care and a fundamental right of a professional.

A changed trend in community care from individual care has given birth to community health nursing. It ranged from speciality hospital, teaching hospital, district hospital, taluk hospital, community health centre, primary health centre and sub centre in the country. Now the nursing care is by the teamwork approach.

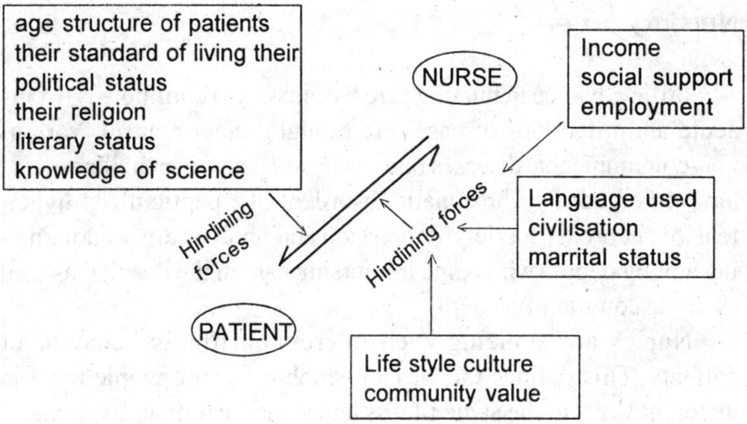

Figure 1.1: Sociological forces in nursing care practices

SOCIOLOGY IN NURSING

There are many seen and unseen utility of knowledge of sociology in nursing. They can be enumerated as under:

- Right of individual is understood
- Responsibility for health increases
- Family pattern influencing health is understandable
- Cultural factors and cultural pattern influencing health and disease is perceived
- Role of social structure is made visible
- Social problems are analysed
- Social agencies that are available becomes visible and taken to help the sick and injured

Practice of nursing is associated with basic and applied sciences that form the pillar of nursing care. But each society has its own religious ideology, tenets and misconception, which are based on the social structure of a community.

Social scientists are helping nursing profession in understanding problems such as the social component of health and diseases, illness behavior, efficient use of technology and to work within the available resources.

A brief account of area of interest for sociology and nursing are given under the following heads;

Nursing care

Scientific advance in nursing care has increased enormously. Many acute and infectious diseases are brought under control. Various non-communicable diseases like cancer, diabetes, mental illness etc., have emerged. Psychosomatic disorders like peptic ulcer, hypertension, neurosis, anxiety, depression and phobias are predominating among people who come for nursing care in the hospital as well as in the community.

Nurses are evincing keen interest on illness behavior of patients. This defines the way in which different people react in different ways to the same illness and same treatment. Even manifestations are different in different personalities. When education and social status are identified as the cause of the difference, the nurse can make out the influence of the sociological predisposing factors in the causation of illness.

Anatomy, physiology, microbiology and pathology are found insufficient in nursing care formulations. The nurses need to be oriented with socio-cultural aspects of illness. Thus nurse has to integrate her nursing clinical knowledge and social knowledge so that she can effectively serve the patient. Thus history, geography, economics, political science, and behavioural sciences are current areas of interest in nursing profession.

Community nursing care

As a community health nurse one has to know why some people accept and some do not accept the given nursing care. In spite of the fact that there is total benefit by the nursing care, there is likelihood of not using the provided service as expected. Available vaccines, available family planning methods, available RCH care services, dietary pattern, child rearing practices, personal hygiene and environmental hygiene etc., need consideration. Community resistance is felt in all spheres of above health care activities. In health care, in nursing care and in welfare activities it is overseen. Social scientists are helping nursing profession to understand the problems in their professional roles and relationships, hospital organisation and team approach. The common theme is human behavior, which needs to be tackled.

EPIDEMIOLOGY

Epidemiologists, who study the determinants and distribution of communicable and non-communicable diseases, are close associates of social scientists in studying the sociological aspect of the nursing profession. The relationship of social factors like income, social class, occupation, housing, overcrowding, customs, habits, values, conventions and other illness behavior in relation to any condition pertaining to health and disease have been justified. In the present social system, there are different attitudes and values in population that influence the sick role. Studying such factors is relavent to nursing profession because the nurse has to play her role in the hospital, in the ward and in the community.

The course of any illness has its own natural history of disease. This is influenced by many structural factors from social strata. The scientific examination of human behavior helps nurse to enhance her skills in promoting health, protecting health and in providing required rehabilitation.

Sociology of nursing profession can be depicted through following diagram:

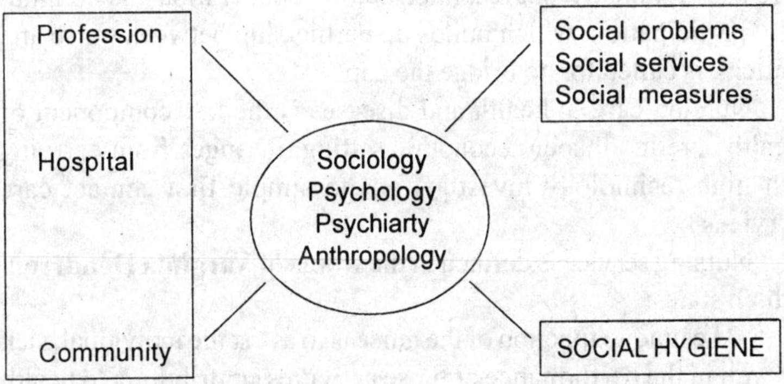

Figure 1.2: Interrelated areas of sociology for nursing care in the community

2

Nursing Profession

Health care and nursing care are influenced by an array of demographic, socioeconomic, political and environmental factors that are constantly changing. Major obstacles to health are poverty and deteriorating economic conditions. The demand for trained nurses has been increasing due to social crises, political crises, aging process of the population and deteriorating environmental factors. Despite improvement in health care, there is a wide gap between health service givers and consumers i.e., nurses and patients; more so between trained nurse and the needy population. Hence effective use of human resource, intersectoral cooperation and community participation, which builds up partnership between nurse and patient, is called for, to bridge the gap.

Nursing care in health and diseases is the key component of health care in all socio economic setting. It ranges from carrying out high technology investigations to simple first contact care services.

Nursing service is defined in the words of **Varginia Hendrson**, which states:

"The unique function of the nurse is to assist the individual, sick or well in the performance of those activities contributing to health or its recovery (or to a peaceful death) that she would perform unaided if she had the necessary strength, will or knowledge and to do this in such a way as to help a patient regain independence as soon as possible".

Functional description of nursing profession is given as under:

Nursing profession help individual, family and group to determine and achieve their physical, mental and social potential in the context of their environment in which they live. It includes; promotion of health and prevent illness. Nursing profession always plans to give:

- Care of the ill
- Rehabilitation of disabled and
- Compassion at dying.

Nursing profession is an art and science, requiring understanding and application of specific knowledge and skills. They are derived from humanities, physical science, social science, medical science, and biological science.

Nursing care covers:

- Managing physical and mental health in health and disease
- Monitoring and ensuring the quality of health care practice
- Organising and managing health care system
- Caring and helping the well, the ill and the dying
- Teaching the art and science of nursing for self care, family guidance
- Advanced educational preparation, coupled with practical experience, enabling nurse to practice at an advanced level
- Innovators and participants in complementary and traditional approaches to health care
- No enforcement of boundaries between professions and even within profession, allow no conflict and no restriction for a better nursing care.

Context of Nursing Profession

Nursing profession is influenced by the context in which it takes place. The force field for nursing practice is illustrated in Figure 2.1.

In the above figure, we observe that economic resource, demography, epidemiology, environment, politics, social factors and cultural factors have shown impact on nursing practice.

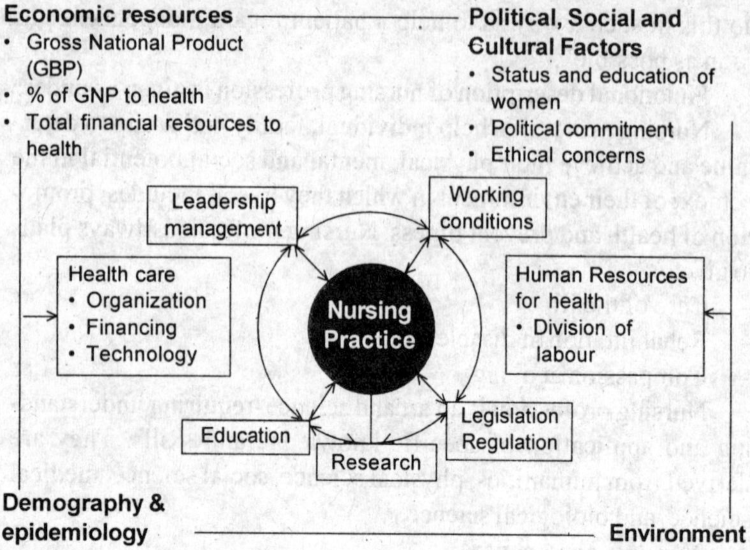

Figure 2.1: Force field for nursing practice

Nursing regulatory body

Nursing practice, nursing education and functioning of health care system under law has come under the governance of a statutory regulatory body called **Nursing Council of India** at national level.

In addition to laying the firm foundation of modern system of nurse training, Florence Nightingale was responsible for the total reorganisation of civil hospitals and military hospitals. She brought out many reformations including improving sanitation and hygiene of Indian army. Her pledge is still vivid even today:

" *I solemnly pledge before God and in the presence of this assembly to pass my life in purity and to practice my profession faithfully. I will abstain from whatever is deleterious and mischievous and will not take or knowingly administer any harmful drug. I will do in all my power to maintain and elevate the standard of my profession and will hold in confidence all personal matters committed to my keeping and all my family affairs coming to my knowledge in the practice of my calling. With loyalty I will endeavour to aid the physician in his work, and devote myself to the welfare of those committed to my care."*

..............*Nightingale pledge*

NURSING ORGANISATION

British Nurse Association was the first organised body of trained nurses in 1887. The Matron of St. Bartholomew's hospital Ms. Gorden Manson was the Founder of this Association. She is popularly known as Mrs. Bedford Fenwick. In 1894, Matron's Council of Great Britain and Matron's Council of Ireland were formed. In 1901 First International Congress of Nurses was held at Buffalo. The professional colleges were started in 1916 and in 1919 **The Nurses Registration Act** was enacted.

In India with establishment of Lady Reading Health School in 1918 preparation of nursing workers started.

The changing trend in the community care, the goal of W.H.O. in Primary Health Care and Health For All made the concept of nursing professional care restructured. Nursing beyond the Year 2000 tried to include the need for continuing assessment of change of nursing care services. Three strategic aims were formulated. which are:

a) A new multisectoral systems approach to health care delivery and full collaboration of health care personnel at all levels
b) A shift in the focus of workforce development in nursing and midwifery to reflect the country's health needs, with particular emphasis on vulnerable groups
c) Revitalisation and reorientation of nursing and midwifery education and practice to meet the challenge of the future.

Nursing profession is enlarging to include mental health nursing, home visiting, occupational health nursing etc., which are of utmost importance in the practice of nursing profession.

Nursing profession holds highest responsibility in discharging 75% of medical, surgical and obstetrical treatment and 100% of community nursing care services. It occupies a strategic position in health care of well and ill and is committed to achieve the goal of **HEALTH FOR ALL.**

Nursing profession has been defined by the American Nurse Association as under;

"A blend of intellectual attainment, attitudes an mental skills based on the principles of scientific medicine acquired by means of a prescribed course in a school of nursing affiliated to a hospital, recognised by the state and practiced in conjunction with curative and preventive medicine by an individual licensed to do so by the state"

Nurse in her nursing profession recognises and understands the fundamental needs of a healthy person or a sick person and knows how these needs can best be met with. She possesses a body of scientific nursing knowledge which is based on science and technology. She will apply this knowledge to an individual and the community. She discerns her area of work with the work of other health professionals.

The term professional nurse is given to those who are graduated as per Nursing Council of India guidelines and affiliated University of Health Sciences.

The characteristics of nursing profession are:

- Mental and physical health
- Alertness
- Technical competence
- Dependability
- Ability to inspire confidence
- Resourcefulness
- Poise
- Consideration for others
- Cooperation
- Agreeableness
- Nursing culture
- Work satisfaction
- Professionally responsible

Professional responsibility of a nurse can be illustrated as (Fig. 2.2):

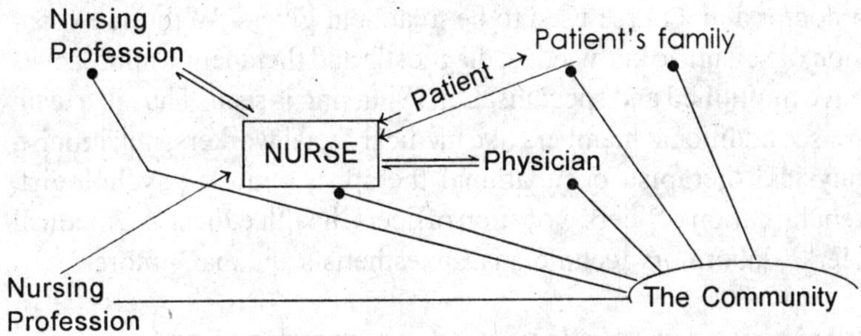

Figure 2.2: Professional responsibility of nurse

Multi Diciplinary Approach

In addition to health sector, all related sectors and aspects of national and community development, in particular agriculture, animal husbandry, food industry, education, housing, public works and communication are to join and give health care through a multidisciplinary approach.

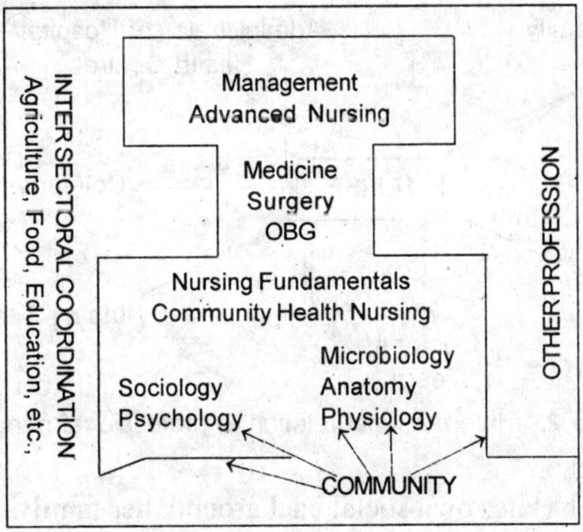

Figure 2.3: Multidisciplinary approach in health care

Team nursing

Very few activities in nursing are carried out in isolation. Most of nursing work is to be done as a teaching process. Centuries ago a doctor and a nurse used to be treatment givers. With the expansion of scientific knowledge, diagnostic and therapeutic approaches have multiplied and specialisation in nursing is seen. Thus in a team we see additional members like medical social workers, nutritionist, physical therapist, occupational therapist, clinical psychologist, rehabilitation officers, vocation officers, health educators, medical clerks, laboratory technicians, anaesthetists and many more.

Interpersonal relations and communication

The effect of patients on each other has received relatively little attention. A patient to be alone is not found beneficial. Nurse and doctor often talk and behave as if each patient were being treated as an isolated and separate individual. They ignore the influence of patients on each other and the influence of nurse on each other. Nursing the whole patient refers to **the patient's body and mind, his or her physical and emotional difficulties** (Fig. 2.4**).**

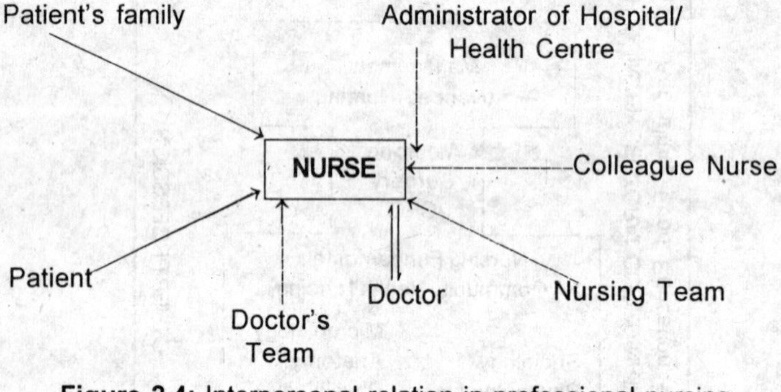

Figure 2.4: Interpersonal relation in professional nursing

A nurse has her own social background, her family, and commitments and is similar to that of a patient and a doctor. Patient's anxiety may be overlooked. Nurses' new social obligations to patients, doctor, administrators may be overlooked. A good culture and good communication is a theme of high quality nursing component.

In case of professional relation with doctors and nurse interrelationship is influenced by anxiety, stress and commitments; with patient relation it is influenced by extent of sickness, sympathy shown to them or physical barrier like hard of hearing in elderly patients and so on.

Principles of nursing profession are highlighted as under:

- *Principles related to meeting the need of patients*
  - Safe and comfortable environment for patient
  - Bed making
  - Admission procedures
  - Observation and charting
  - After receipt of instructions in ward rounds, sound planning of nursing care
  - Discharge procedures
- *Principles of daily fundamental care*
  - Comfort position
  - Care of the skin
  - Care of nails
  - Care of hair
  - Care of mouth
  - Food requirement in terms of balanced diet or therapeutic adaptation of normal diet
  - Elimination and treatment of large intestine
  - Elimination and treatment of bladder
- *Principles to vital signs*
  - Temperature recording and treatment
  - Pulse and B P recording
  - Respiration and nursing treatment of respiratory tract
- *Principles of drug administration*
  - Oral medicine
  - Injections
  - Infusions
  - Transfusions
  - Radiation (X-ray, Cobalt)
- *Principles of therapeutic measures and diagnostic tests*
  - Heat application and withdrawal
  - Treatment of vaginal canal

- Treatment of eye
- Treatment of ear, nose, throat
- Treatment of stomach
- Diagnostic tests

- *Principles of meeting the need of special patients*
  - Infectious diseases
  - Surgery and post surgery
  - Wound bandaging and care
  - Chronic ill patient
  - Care of dying and dead.

The Patient-Recipient of Nursing Care

Man is a biopsychosocial being and understanding him in his environment is utmost important for an effective treatment. Apart from health need, other aspects of needs (human needs) are to be contemplated in diagnosis, therapy and rehabilitation of a given patient. Following different situations (personalities) are encountered that need elucidation.

Infancy

He is completely a helpless patient. He has only reflexes and no activity can be carried out. He is totally dependent for everything. Breast-feeding by mother is an added compliment, which the nursing component should look for. Another point of consideration is to look into growth and development at hospital admission. Because the infant cannot express in terms of adult concepts, it must be assumed that her early experiences are Recalled in the realm of feeling.

Early childhood

A great deal of success in the case management depends on the mother's skill in giving hand with nursing care. Again growth and development, importance of breast feeding are to be considered in analysis of the case. Toilet training, family closeness, play therapy are to be included in the nursing component of health and nursing care.

School age child

School age children always want to conform. They do not know what is expected of them. They have to be informed and even if they know would have forgotten. Hence they need to be reminded and this could help in correcting their behaviour.

Adolescence

They do not have their own identity. They prefer to be known by their own identity than with others. They will imbibe parental values in their opinion. Nursing component is to accept antithetical mannerism, habit of this group of patients.

Adult

It is possible to widen the scope for emotion and to feel strongly about patient's feelings and causes as well as about people.

Old age

Physical disabilities like eyesight and hearing loss should be remembered in this category of patient for an appropriatc action through nursing component. Emotional components like loneliness, worrics, and anxiety are to be taken note in problem evaluation. Recently Geriatric nursing is becoming a speciality.

ILLNESS AND SICK ROLE

Illness is an unwelcome intrusion; while some may regard this as a challenge, many peoples' attitude to illness is much less constructive, and many nursing problems arise because sick people often behave not as adults but as if they were much younger. Under stress they revert to earlier pattern of behaviour (Regress). It is not uncommon for people to adopt this attitude of guilt and shame towards their own suffering. It is interesting to note that word PAIN has come from Greek work POINE, which means penalty. Some of the diseases attract negative attitude by the attending health professional. STD, HIV, AIDS, Leprosy, Tuberculosis are such conditions in the practice of nursing care.

Some patients turn to God and derive comfort from such an action.

Whatever illness people suffer from, at treatment, patient (sick) must give up oneself and submit to the authority of nurses. In some respect sick resembles that of a child who needs attention from his/her mother.

Nursing profession should visualise *attention-seeking behaviour* of patient.

Coping Strategies by the Sick

Hostility

Hostile attitude of the sick is a deterrent to all nursing care unless it is tackled in the beginning itself. Non-cooperative and non-submissive takes away nurses' energy in diagnosis, treatment and rehabilitation. Sympathy, understanding, and taking the help of members of patients' family are available techniques in such cases. Only in case of life saving situations force can be used with ward boys, which in no way is inhuman.

Manipulation

In communication, progress response and in nursing examination, patient may show manipulated tactics. Manipulation is highly dangerous because of its negative influence in problem solving through data collection, analysis and assessment. Second opinion, re examination and repeat assessment is available means to overcome manipulation.

Loneliness

This is natural in case of geriatric patients and in them it is reversible with available means of showing concern, sympathy, constant listening to their complaints and psychotherapy. There are selected group of patients who are basically introvert who are not to be confused with loneliness. Good interaction, assurance and building confidence helps in overcoming loneliness due to their introvert nature.

Rehabilitation

It is an element of social integration with physiotherapy, occupational therapy, speech therapy, psychotherapy, educating social welfare work, vocational guidance and placement services. The main aims in rehabilitation are:

- Restoration of function (medical)
- Restore capacity of earning (vocational)
- Restore social relation (social)
- Restore confidence (psychological).

Illness and disability are a threat to economic security and involve more suffering than pain connected with illness. Worry over finance, disrupted family relation, unemployment, loss of organ etc., not only delay recovery but also healing of organic lesion.

Nursing profession should have a sufficient knowledge of the community resources to enable them to advice the patient and his family.

Their burden will be lightened if specialists in social work and vocational guidance also participate in patients' care. The team required for rehabilitations is:

- Orthopaedician
- Physiotherapist
- Occupational therapist
- Speech therapist
- Audiologist
- Psychologist
- Psychosocial counsellor
- Social worker
- Government administrators.

Nursing responsibility, as a professional is a wider activity in collaboration with team suggested above; she follows instruction, monitors rehabilitation, records the progress of action and submits report of progress to concerned specialists of rehabilitation team.

Since nursing element is a chemical bond in each act of rehabilitation be it physical, vocational, social or psychological, no specific delineation can be done as to nursing responsibility. Nurse initiates, implements, monitors, and reports and dismisses and thus she is the key person in nursing care services.

3

Nurse and The Hospital

Hospitals work on socioeconomic and political framework of society. The word *Hospes* is a root word for hospital (even for Hotel and Hospice) which originally was shelter of the homeless and for entertainment of travellers. In modern times, however, the chief function of the hospital has been the care and treatment of the sick. Hospital of the future would extend the care of the sick with in its walls to the nursing supervision and nursing care of the sick within a given district served by the hospital. Presently they have OPD, IPD, care of the ambulatory sick on emergency and now concept of Home care programme for the sick extending from the hospital is being perceived seen. Responsibility of the hospital is fixed for the realisation of community health programmes and physician, nurse, dietician, social worker, physiotherapist, administrators are taught in the hospital. While the education of health workers and health professionals are prime concern, Research and its application within the hospital is time tested and reliable.

HOSPITAL SOCIOLOGY

Hospital is a social organisation which gives medical care for the society. Doctors are service givers whereas patients are consumers.

Apart from medical care teaching, training and research are undertaken. This is coordinated by different professional which include medical, nursing, Para medical etc.

Staff relations, emotional atmosphere, development of new diagnostic and therapeutic lines of management have influenced social dynamics of the hospital.

Social aspects of sick role, nurse patient relationship and doctor nurse relationship have impact on the medical care utilization.

Types of Hospitals:

Table 3.1: Types of hospital

Public Health Sector	**Private Sector**	**Indigenous Systems of Medicine**
Teaching hospitals attached to medical colleges Civil hospitals (District hospitals) ESI hospitals CGHS hospitals Defence hospitals Railway hospitals	Private hospitals Nursing homes	Ayurveda hospitals Sidda hospitals Unani hospitals Homoeopathy hospitals Naturopathy Yoga hospital

Hospital Standardisation

Hospital construction, organisation and practice that serve as standards have been recommended from time to time. Hospital administrators, physicians, nurses, dieticians and other health workers have to thrive hard for establishing standards. Minimum standards for hospitals can classify them under fully approved, provisionally approved or not approved. These formulations depend on the nature of hospital administration by the existing administrators.

Evaluation of hospital is done by periodic assessment and medical auditing. It is reflected on mortality rate and hospital bed occupancy.

HOSPITAL ORGANISATION

In a hospital there will be visiting Board of Directors who direct the administrators. Usual pattern consists of units, departments and sections which can be represented in Fig. 3.1.

Function of a hospital is unique in human service through medical care, nursing care, surgical intervention, emergency care, preventive care and rehabilitation care for the public.

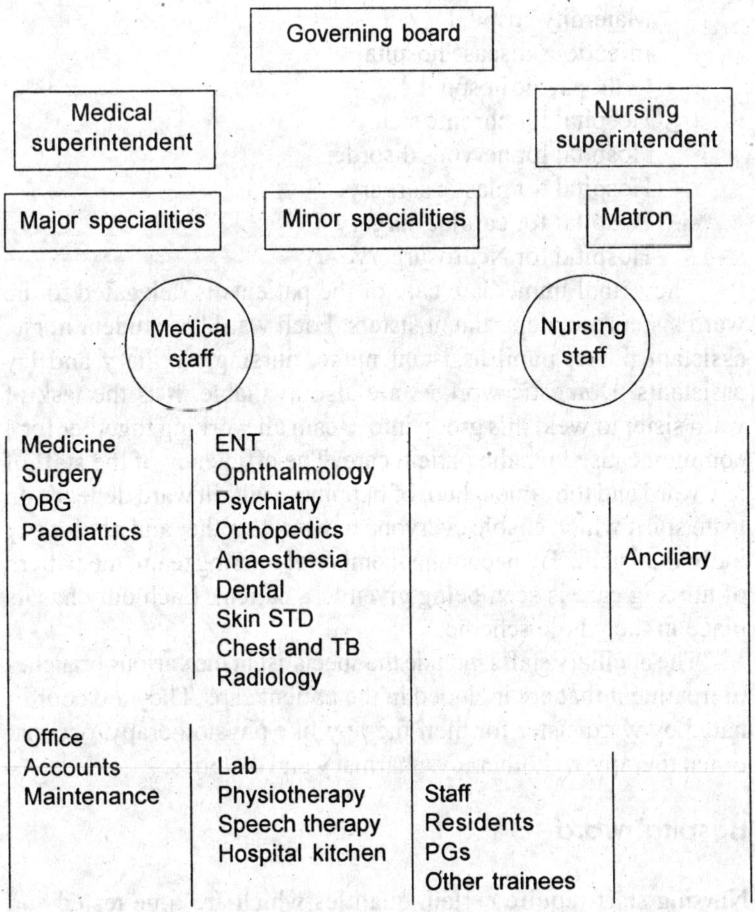

Figure 3.1: Organisation of a hospital

Students may pay a fee to hospital for its use as a practice field or the hospital may pay the student for his/her service during learning period. If a student is a paid member, hospital can demand a reasonably high standard of performance and conformity to hospital regulations.

Till 1950, all general hospitals were treating both general and varied cases. Tuberculosis hospitals (sanatoria) were more in number. Some of the recent introductions of hospitals are:

- General hospital
- Children hospital
- Maternity hospital
- Infectious disease hospital
- Orthopaedic hospital
- Hospital for chronic sick
- Hospital for nervous disorder
- Hospital for plastic surgery
- Hospital for cardiac surgery
- Hospital for Neurosurgery.

The actual immediate care of the patients is delegated to the ward sisters and department sisters. Each ward has student nurse, assistant nurse, pupil assistant nurse, nursing auxiliary and lay assistants. Domestic workers are also available. It is the task of ward sister to weld this group into a team all working together for a common cause viz., the patient care. The efficiency of the staff of any ward and the atmosphere of happiness within ward depends on team spirit which enable everyone to work together and not for any individual gain. By becoming member of nursing team, the pattern of nursing care is seen being given to a patient. Each duty has its place in the whole scheme.

The ancillary staffs include the specialist in the various branches of treatment that are included in the patient care. They are coordinated by ward sister for their therapy like physiotherapy, occupational therapy, radiotherapy, pharmacy and dietetics.

Hospital ward

Nursing staff require certain qualities which are time tested and remunerative from humanitarian angle. They are:

- Patience, sympathy, understanding
- Gentleness and willingness
- Reliability
- Resourcefulness
- Power of observation.

Duties of a Nurse

The requirements towards patient

- Rest
- Toilet
- Diet
- Excretion of waste material
- Mental outlook

The requirements towards doctor

- Carrying out instruction and written report, avoids risk of omissions
- Nature of sleep
- Pain relief activity

The requirements for self

- Cleanliness
- Clothing
- Food
- Rest and exercise.

Consumer Protection Act on Nursing

One who purchases nursing service for his or her use is called consumer. The user of nursing service with permission is also a consumer as per legal terminology.

Nursing service should be given free from defects, deficiencies and free from unfair practices. Receipts, bills, cash memo against all services are compulsory as per the Act. Consumer can demand good services in exchange of money. The Consumer Protection Act of 1986 ensures rights covering all nursing services in hospitals, nursing homes, clinic, cooperative clinics and consultation centres.

All consumers are becoming knowledgeable about disease, health care and complications. They are assertive about their rights to competent and prudent care and their right to privacy of information. Easy access to information in internet has lead to more health care standards and health policies. Most of the consumer groups, consumer committees, consumer forum have active consumers who can regulate political actions on health care delivery system.

Nursing education is affected with serious medical errors. Deaths and lawsuits with high associated costs are increasing with these errors. This is influencing the need for improving the quality of health care in India. Majority of errors are attributed to nursing profession and therefore, nursing faculty and nursing administrators are increasingly concerned with ensuring true competence of nurse student and nursing faculty. Shortage of nurses and quality teaching and training of nurses in the country is being more and more realised.

Consumer courts set up under COPRA at National, State and District level provide simple, inexpensive and speedy redressal of consumer disputes including excess price charged. Complaints can be made for compensation on a plain paper without court fee and without a lawyer.

District Forum can be approached for compensation up to 5 lakhs; the State commission should be approached if it is in the range of 5 to 20 lakhs. The Department of Consumer Affairs under the Central Ministry of Government of India is in charge of the above.

Following factors are taken note of under Consumer Protection Act:

- Consumer health awareness
- Existing constraints in the infrastructure
- Misuse by the consumer
- Safeguard of nursing service providers.

Nursing education has to adopt competency based education and performance assessment in nursing colleges as part of annual evaluations and accreditation. The primary focus should be a harmony between doctor and nurse to promote patient safety and to reduce errors in all walks of nursing care.

Sociology of health problems

The management of patient require appropriate, timely and on the spot decisions. Planning patients' care should consider each patient's condition and each patient's unique problem. This is important in healing touch of the patient which can be called social therapy.

On many occasions patient may need counselling on his illness or disease condition. The given case may be acutely ill, chronically ill or apparently healthy. An understanding of the patient's condition helps in giving priority and personal touch during the treatment schedule.

Health problems are often associated with social problems, which need tackling through social therapy and counselling. Invasive interventions need informed consent and treatment under supervision, which any common man expects.

4 Nurse and The Community

Progress of nursing has reflected the social outlook of present century, so also health centres, hospitals, district hospitals and teaching hospitals.

In the beginning nurse has to adjust, at her entry, to new surroundings and should not get bewildered by many aspect of hospital life. Preconceived idea by a nursing student about hospital and about nursing may bear little resemblance to reality; hence the need of understanding of structure and function of hospital which highlight the social structure of the organisation.

Nursing care is a continuous exercise to be carried out day and night without interruption, for the sick there is no time interval. Nursing staff is geared to serve the sick. All disciplines like dispensary, laboratory, X-ray, physiotherapy and ancillary staff like orderly, porter, domestic workers and so on have to work diligently in the serving of the sick. Hospital is a complex organisation and demands the attention that is not equalled in many other spheres.

Nursing profession has a greater role to play not only in curative treatment of disease but also to restore the patient as far as possible to full activity. The cooperation of patient is required so that he can play his part in recovery and subsequent welfare. Nurse is responsible in getting the full cooperation of the patient.

Nursing has its role in hospital research. Experience and observation has helped health staff to give a confidence based specific treatment. Joseph Lister's "anti septic surgery" has opened the door to great surgical advances. Such great examples are available to mitigate sufferings of mankind and truely are part of hospital services.

Malthusian Theory of Population Explosion

This theory postulates that over population is controlled by natural calamities like volcano, earthquake, floods, epidemics, etc. Though it is not a scientific version it can only be an antithesis of population.

Effects of Overpopulation

Impact of overpopulation on the society is many. Major effects noticeable are hindrance to national development, unemployment, illiteracy, poor housing, non-availability of health care facility, poor environmental sanitation and fast development of slums and shantytowns as its consequences.

National Population Policy

To achieve National Demographic goals, India developed National population policy in 1976, modified in 1977 and restructured in 2000. The National population policy of 2000 has laid emphasis on women's education, child survival, unmet needs of family planning, coverage of under-served population, adolescent health and education and participation of men in Planned Parenthood. Following are the demographic goals of NPP by 2010:

1. Service, supply and infrastructure for unmet needs of RCH.
2. Free and compulsory education up to 14 years of age and school dropout reduced to below 20%.
3. IMR to 30 per 1000 live births
4. MMR to 1 per 1000 live births
5. 100% coverage of UIP.
6. Age at marriage for girls 18 years.
7. 100% deliveries by trained persons.
8. Cafeteria approach of family planning methods.

9. Registration of vital events 100%.
10. Integrated approach for RTI and STD.
11. Control of communicable disease by priority.
12. Integration and availability of Indian system of medicine for RCH care and home visiting.
13. Total fertility rate is brought down to replacement level by 2010 by promoting small family norm.
14. F.P. is made as family welfare and as a people centred programme. National Population Policy implemented through Zilla Parishad and DH and FW office. Fully implemented NPP can reduce global population, crude birth rate, IMR and Total Fertility Rate. This also envisages unmet need of contraceptive services in the community.

National Family Planning Programme (NFPP)

In 1952 India launched FP programme. The approach is "Extension Education Approach" for motivating people to accept small family norm. Since 1965 to 1970 IUD (Lippes loop) made a mark in F.P. programme. Later Copper-T was used under National F.P. programme. In 1966 Ministry of Health got bifurcated to Health and F.P. Wings. The infrastructure of F.P. was strengthened. In every 5 years plan, top priority is being given to F.P.

PPC in 1970 and MTP in 1971 were added as additional forces in Family Planning. National Population Policy gave vivid picture for action in 1976.

In 1977 F.P. was renamed as Family Welfare Planning since it involved family welfare activities.

Primary health care approach, Health For All approach, long term demographic goal of Net Reproduction Rate 1 by 2007 which imply 2 child family norm, goal of Birth Rate 21, goal of Death Rate 9 and Couple Protection Rate of 60% are strategic phenomena under NFPP in India.

Seventh Five Year Plan incorporated UIP, ORT (under CSSM) under F.W. planning. (Universal Immunisation Programme, Oral Rehydration Therapy, Child Survival and Safe Motherhood).

Since 1997 we have unified R.C.H. (Reproductive and Child Health) integrated with Eighth Five-Year Plan for need based, client oriented service.

In the year 2000, Government of India reinforced the comprehensive National Population Policy.

Financial allocation to FWP is better reviewed by following table:

Table 4.1: Financial allocation to FWP

Year	Expenditure
First 5 year plan	0.65 crore
Fifth 5 year plan	285.60 crores
Eighth 5 year plan	6195.00 crores
Ninth 5 year plan	58920.30 crores
Tenth 5 year plan	27125.00 crores
Eleventh 5 year plan	136147.00 crores

Nurses and Patient

A somewhat sobering statement, which is worth careful consideration, is "Do the sick no harm". This is from none other than Florence Nightingale. Constant vigilance is needed in nursing procedures in order that these may be carried out with the highest degree of competence.

Checking administration of dangerous drugs, measures to prevent cross infection, care of elderly, care of child, care of women in labour need substantial attention, which are available only from nursing profession.

Anxiety and stress of patient need attention to overcome distressing effect on family life. To watch an experienced and sympathetic ward sister set about the task of allaying the fears of anxious relatives and establishing their confidence in the hospital and the staff is a most valuable lesson in good human relationship.

Nursing Ethics

It is the code of moral behavior and rules of conduct related to nursing. Compassion, sympathy, pleasant manner are required for successful management of cases.

Loyalty and obedience to authorities, recognition of experience of senior staff, maintaining confidentiality on affairs of patient are other aspect of ethical issues.

Trustworthiness and reliability are essential if the nurse is to develop a sense of responsibility as a member of nursing team.

It is the moral and ethical obligation of a nursing profession to offer one's service to a patient irrespective of social distinction, race, creed or caste.

Professional Etiquette

Certain rules of behavior for maintaining discipline and orderliness, which are necessary for safety and welfare of patient is of prime importance.

While, nursing staff are addressed with a title of matron, sister nurse etc., patient should be identified by their name and not by number or disease. Courtesies to visitors who visit their patients, improve patient-nurse relationship and this extends to the good hospital environment. Courtesy shown to seniors matters much in nursing profession etiquette.

Major principles of nursing ethics

(i) Principles of doing good *(Beneficence)*
(ii) Serve the ill with fairness, equity and impartially *(Justice)*
(iii) Patient can choose his choice of treatment *(Respect for autonomy)*
(iv) Principles of not harming patient (*Non maleficence*).

Formal procedure in nursing ethics

Values and norms drawn are followed and ethical issues are considered while attending formal procedures in the following:

- Organ donation
- Dealing with human life e.g.,, M.T.P.
- Living will
- Advanced life directives in terminally ill and cancer patient
- Dying declaration.

Professional nursing ethics

There are certain moral principles, which guide nursing profession in day-to-day interaction with colleagues, patients, and relatives of patient. They are:

Contract

Fully attending till normalcy is an utmost requirement when patients are attended. It is the courtesy required in the community. When a case is being handled, one has entered into a contract with patient to do all required professional act to bring him back to normal and not disallowing in the middle. It will become breech of contract.

Confidentiality

In the nursing profession it is obligatory to maintain strictly confidentiality about the physical and mental status of a patient.

Rationale use of drugs

In nursing profession, need for use of discretion is very critical in administering the right dosage in right time and of required combination in order to relieve the patient's suffering or to avoid any distress and / or help the patient's speedy recovery.

No over-investigation

Unnecessary investigation, which might bring discomfort to the patient and/or result in unnecessary expenditure, should be avoided.

Animal experiment

Humaneness and animal ethical procedures are followed in research drug trial etc.

Patient related ethics in the community

They are guiding principles for nursing profession, which involve:

- Compassion
- Confidentiality
- Element of informed consent
- Obligation to treat
- Respect for person
- Solidarity
- Well being or beneficence.

Community Development Programme (CDP)

Community Development is a process designed to create conditions of economic and social progress for the whole community with its active participation and the fullest possible reliance upon the community's initiative. Here people are brought together for their development.

C.D.P. was launched in 1952 for the all round development of Rural areas. It is an organised programme by community development blocks, each covering 1,20,000 population. There are about 6100 community development blocks in the country.

It envisages following programmes:

a. Improvement of agriculture
b. Improvement of communication
c. Education
d. Health
e. Sanitation
f. Housing

The community development block will work for intensive development for 5 years followed by continued work in second phase of 5 years. It is mainly centrally sponsored programme. By its programme, it is tackling rural poverty and unemployment.

Panchayat Raj System

It is a 3-tier health system at 3 levels they are:

- *Panchayat* at village level
- *Panchayat samiti* at Block level
- *Zilla parishad* at district level

Panchayat at Village Level

Gram Panchayat is an executive organ responsible for village development. It has a president (*Sarpanch*), vice president, a secretary. Administration, sanitation, public health, socioeconomic development are included. When they give legal verdict it is called *Nyaya Panchayat*.

Panchayat Samiti at Block Level

About 100 villages of 1,00,000 population has a *samiti* consisting of *sarpanchs* of the block. B.D.O. acts as secretary of *samiti*. It is responsible for community development programme of the block.

Zilla Parishad at District Level

It is rural local self Government of the district. All heads of *panchayat samiti* are members. Deputy Commissioner (Collector) is a non-voting member. It will have above 60 members. Health services, Family planning service of the district come under *Zilla Parishad*.

Communication

"It is a two way process of exchanging and shaping ideas, feelings and message."

Communication can be for:

- Acquiring knowledge

– Learning skills
– Develop good attitude

Day-to-day communications are going on in social life. Components of communication are represented as under:

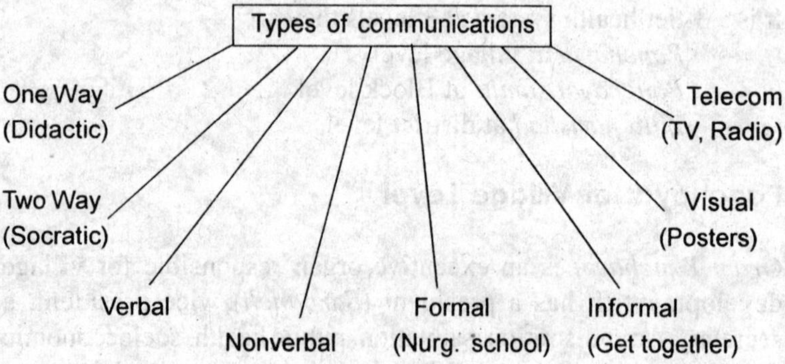

Figure 4.1: Types of communication

VOLUNTARY HEALTH ORGANISATIONS

Promoting the health and welfare of the people has been the motto by some as individual or as a group is known from *vedic* period. This needs a dynamic group and a good social interaction on the part of the group. Nurse as a member of community Health team need orientation and information on such agencies, which are helping human community by their welfare programmes. It is voluntary agencies that have pioneered the health development in any country. They have missionary zeal and an organisation by itself consisting of an administrative body, a committee to raise funds through membership and all actions are through voluntary basis.

According to Gunn and Platt, Voluntary Health Agencies have certain characteristics. They are enumerated as under:

- They are organised.
- Have an autonomous board.
- Holds meeting.
- Collect fund.
- Conduct Public Health Programme.

- Create Health awareness.
- Help in policy making.
- They are small enough to reach any place.

After independence, India has seen well-developed network of voluntary health associations, which functioned for the welfare of mankind. Major agencies, which are worth mentioning, are under following heads:

1. ***Relief operation***
   Indian Red Cross Society
   Bharath Sevak Samaj
   All India Blind Relief Society
2. ***Specific Disease control***
   Hind Kusht Nivaran Sangh
   Tuberculosis Association of India
   Indian Cancer Society
3. ***R.C.H.***
   Indian Council of Child Welfare
   The *Kasturba* Memorial Fund
   F.P.A.I.
   All India Women's Conference
4. ***Professional bodies***
   The Trained Nurses' Association
   I.M.A
   Indian Dental Association
   General Practitioners' Association
5. ***Social welfare***
   Central Social Welfare Board
   State Social Welfare Board

General functions of voluntary Health agencies in India

- Medical Relief
- Initiation of measures according to their objectives
- Supplementing Government effort
- Development of manpower, media and methods for Health Education
- Evaluation of Health activities in India.

5

Social Sciences and Behavioural Sciences

Without sociological aspect and social content, health is almost incomplete. Diagnosis, investigation and treatment are influenced by social factors and economic factors. Literacy, sanitation, nutrition, culture and behaviour predispose to diseases and disorders.

Interrelated areas are grouped and depicted in a diagram as under:

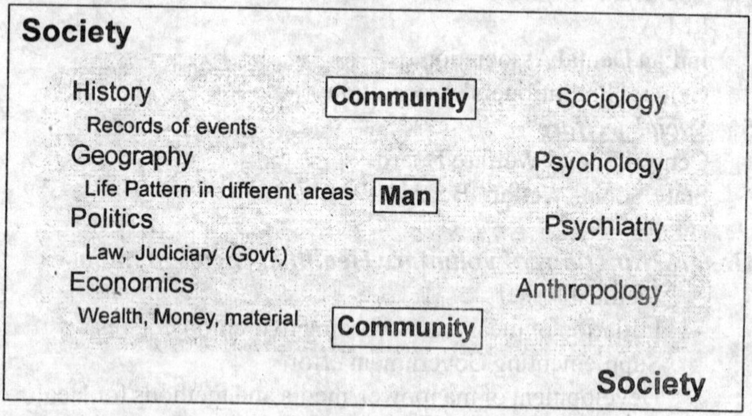

Figure 5.1: Social sciences and behavioural sciences in health and disease

Definitions/Commonly Used Sociological Terms

Medicosocial:
Study of cultural factors and social relations in connection with illness and social principles in medical organisation and treatment

Sociology:
Study of human relationship and human behaviour for better understanding of the pattern of human life

Social structure (Social anatomy):
Knowledge of the structure of the society or particular community (age, sex, housing, social group, economics)

Social function (Social physiology):
The way society functions as an organised unit

Social problems (Social pathology):
Systematic study of relation between human disease and social condition

Social management (Social therapy):
Social and political action for betterment of the condition

Social follow up (Social post mortem):
Ultimate or remote cause of disease

Social factors:
It is a sequence of interaction between human beings and the effect of the action of individuals on one another and of their joint action e.g., occupation, income, social class, education, marital status, rural urban area

Marriage:
A condition of man and woman legally united for the purpose of living together and procreating lawful offspring

Family:
A group related by blood, marriage, or by adoption, living together and eating from common kitchen and spending money from common purse

Stages of family:
Formation — Growth — Retraction — Disintegration

Types of family:
Nuclear, Joint, Extended, Three generation, Stem matriarchal, Problem, Broken, Quise

Problem family:
Where members are unable to discharge or prevented from discharging minimum family responsibilities

Broken family:
Where father or mother or both are absent on account of disease, deficiency, destitution, dependence, despondency, delinquency or degeneracy.

Quise family:
Family of homosexual

Matrifocal family:
Mother and children (husband deceased)

Culture:
Learned behaviour, which has been socially acquired

Cultural factor:
Religion, custom, habit, attitude, tradition and belief

Religion:
Ways of classification of human into various groups like Hindu, Muslim, Christian, Jews and Parsee

Habit:
It is an acquired faculty to act in a certain manner, without reason and deliberation or thought

***Attitude*:**
Mental habit acquired from social experience that predisposes as to specific objects, persons or situation in a definite way

Tradition:
Set of rules associated with strict sanction that act as guide to conduct and tend to produce conformity in a community

Belief:
Things derived from parents, grand parents and other people, which are accepted without trying them to prove they are true

Poverty line:
According to Planning Commission report poverty line refers to:
- Urban area - per capita income below 75 rupees or consuming less than 2100 Kcal diet
- Rural area - per capita income below 65 rupees or consuming less than 2400 Kcal diet

Common Examples of Cultural Practices (In Relation to Health and Disease)

<u>Belief</u>

Definition
Things derived from parents, grand parents and other people, which are accepted without trying them to prove they are true

Examples
1. Certain diseases are due to wrath of God and Goddess and administration of drugs is harmful e.g., chickenpox, measles, mumps
2. STD (VD) is due to sex with women of lower caste or during menses

3. Due to the sin committed in the past life e.g., Tuberculosis, Leprosy
4. Spirit of ghost e.g., hysteria, epilepsy
5. Impure blood e.g., skin diseases, boils, which need purification by taking caster oil or eating *neem* leaves
6. Effect of cold and heat e.g., running nose, reddening of eyes, fisherman foot, angular stomatitis, burning during micturition, heart burn
7. God is present and he is watching all of us over our bad deeds
8. Addition of little water to milk before boiling allow good yield of milk in cows
9. Eating papaya during pregnancy causes abortion
10. Eating green leafy vegetables cause dark skin in growing foetus, if eaten during pregnancy
11. Eating from common plate and drinking from common glass are signs of brotherhood.

Custom

Definition

It is the transmission of a way of doing. By tradition is meant the transmission of a way of thinking or believing (Ross).

Examples

1. Open land is meant for field defecation
2. Latrine within the house is dirty and objectionable
3. Apply cow dung to the floor before religious function
4. Taking bath before food
5. Preventing women performing religious function and forbidding entry to kitchen during menses period
6. Walk bare foot within the house and in the temple
7. Throwing waste outside the house through window
8. Using pond water for human bath, animal bath and cloth wash
9. Holy dip in river during pilgrimage and bringing the same water as holy water to keep at home
10 Keeping the animal within the house
11. White washing house on all festivals
12. Hindus are vegetarians

13. Onion and garlic are not eaten by upper caste people
14. Observing fasting on holy days
15. Prolonged breast-feeding of baby by lactating mother even up to 1 1/2 years
16. No colostrum is given to the newborn
17. *Janam gutti*, honey, cows urine, sugar water are given as first feed to the newborn baby
18. Branding of skin, oil bath once a week, oil application to the head of the child (anterior fontanelle)
19. Smoking with burning side inside the mouth
20. Hubble bubble to all invited guests in the house
21. Wearing *burkha* and *parda*
22. Circumcision among Muslim community
23. Thread ceremony among Hindus
24. *Annaprashana* at one-year age for the child
25. Covering their head by women when they come outside the house or when they participate in family functions with men.

Habits:

Definition

It is an acquired faculty to act in certain manner, without reason and deliberation or thought.

Examples

1. Putting finger in nose, ear
2. Putting sticks in mouth
3. Nail biting
4. Eating fish, egg as hot foods
5. Eating curds, milk, vegetables like cucumber as cold food
6. Alcohol consumption by higher-class society
7. *Ganja, Bhung, Charas* among *Sadhus*
8. Eating pan tobacco with lime and smoking
9. Exchange of cloths in hostel life
10. Applying *kajal* to the eyes
11. Applying *kajal* to the cheek of kids
12. Charcoal, *neem* twig tooth brush in the morning
13. Hand washing after defecation and before eating food

14. Application of turmeric powder before bath by women
15. Walking barefoot
16. Sleeping on the floor.

Tradition

Definition

Sets of rule associated with strict sanction that act as guide to conduct and tend to produce conformity in a community.

Examples

1. Men eat first and women in the last
2. Motherhood respecting religious function during first pregnancy
3. Sending women for first delivery in their parents house
4. Touching the feet of elders to get their wishes
5. Purifying bath before religious function
6. Keeping delivered women away from *pooja* room and kitchen for 10 days and allowing entry after 11th day purifying bath
7. Delivery by the Traditional Birth Attendant
8. Performing marriages within same caste and race
9. Marriage is performed in girls' house
10. Household articles are given at send off to husband's house after marriage
11. Wishful gift given at housewarming ceremony
12. Puncturing ear, nose
13. Offering *pan supari* after food in all social gathering
14. Shaving is done outside house by a barber
15. Taking bath after attending funeral ceremony
16. Performing functions like naming ceremony, birthdays, and anniversaries
17. Child marriage as in *Rajasthanis and* tribal
18. Polygamy, Polyandry as in *Himachala Pradesh adivasis.*

Social sciences like history, economics influence society in general, where as behavioural sciences influence the human behaviour, which is the scientific examination of human behaviour.

Economic

This discipline is very close to Social aspect in a society. Production, distribution, consumption, ownership of material, of goods and of services is dealt in this discipline. Human relation is influenced by economic status of an individual, a family or the society.

History, Geography and Political Science

History and geography deal with the historical aspect and natural worldly atmosphere where animal and man live (biosphere). Economics specify the money, material and manpower in terms of production, distribution and consumption of human resources. Nearly 50% of sociology of nursing profession is contributed by economics, which need underlying. Politics help in formulating laws related to society and its institutions. Thus system of law and system of institution constitute political sciences.

Other Social Sciences

Better understanding of human life and human relationships are understood by sociology. Perception, thought, opinions is all from psychology. Physical, social and cultural history of man is traced by anthropology. Human mental illness is managed by the intervention through psychiatry.

Understanding of sociology, psychology, psychiatry and anthropology have given rise to better understanding and better management of illness in the community. They also deal with social problems, social measures, social security and social hygiene which are utmost important in day-to-day management of human illness and maintenance of positive health of the community.

Socio Demographic Impact on Nursing

The socio demographic process still remains elusive. The development of the individual as a nurse to be socialised into the profession requires her to understand the interlocking communication relative concepts, unknown relationships, newer ideas, rules and regulations of the society. She has to account for present, past and future of the nursing care given to the society.

Nursing science require organisational culture through socialisation within nursing profession. Social change in our society should get imbibed in the nursing profession for needed social adjustments of nurses. The social change makes the profession to think in terms of the following set up:

Above items may not directly mean norms, beliefs, and values but set the nurse as a free will human being within the network of entirety. This describes the agents of socialisation within the nursing profession. The role of mutual interaction between nurse and nurse; nurse and doctor and nurse and patient has been found effective.

Many things have changed since Nightingale's era; what remains, however, is the need of a key understanding about human beings as individuals and their placement in a comprehensive social framework.

Health, Single family, joint family, extended family, ethnic groups, religious groups do make an impact on the emotional and financial needs of the individual in times of crisis. Professional nurse is to provide care to persons of various social groups who have different values, beliefs and perceptions of health and illness.

Indian society is mainly rural in nature constituting 78% of population. There are about 7,00,000 villages and each village is with a population of 500 to 2000. Large, dense and permanent settlement form urban area, accounts for 22% of population. According to 2001 census there are 8637 towns and cities. Now there are 300 mega cities indicating extent of urbanisation. We come across occupational diversity and impersonal social life.

Nursing profession has a crucial role to play in helping the country to achieve demographic goals of National Population Policy by 2010, which are as under:

1) Service, supply and infrastructure for unmet needs of RCH
2) Free and compulsory education up to 14 years of age and school drop out reduced to below 20%
3) IMR to 30 per 1000 live births
4) MMR to 1 per 1000 live births
5) 100 percent coverage of U I P
6) Age at marriage for girls 18 years
7) 100% deliveries by trained persons
8) Cafeteria approach of family planning methods
9) Registration of vital events 100%
10) Integrated approach for RTI and STD
11) Control of communicable disease by priority
12) Integration and availability of Indian system of medicine for RCH care and home visiting
13) Total fertility rate is brought to replacement level by 2010 by promoting small family norm
14) Family planning is made as family welfare and as a people centered programme.

Cultural Pattern on Nursing

Culture is defined as values, ceremonies and ways of life characteristic of a given social group. Culture is one of the most distinctive properties of human social association. Culture stands for mode of living, language, custom and belief. Hence it is socially acquired and learned behaviour.

Economic status and social changes has a direct impact on one's life style and living conditions. Low economic status, poor standard of living and low per capita income result in poor health conditions. Any Economic Policy of a country will influence the trend in economic development of a country and in turn the most crucial component namely health care policy, health care delivery, Medicare, social security and education. These changes in trends have relevance to the nursing education. Affordability of a patient has a major influence on nursing component in Health Care Delivery System. Hence, nursing component has to respond to these modalities in her therapeutic relationship and nursing care.

Nurse has to adopt herself to the position of current health care professional with the economic challenges in nursing care. Hospitals may combine non-nursing resources with limited nursing resources to decrease the total costs of services. Hence a nurse is at pressure to excel her clinical resources management and to design care delivery that provides a less costly service that satisfies the customer requirements.

Coordinated care by a nurse reduces wastage of limited health care resources. Hospital care is costlier than home based or clinic based care, which needs a nurse to understand financial and resource management and leadership role to ensure the effective and efficient use of resources. Most appropriate level of care and most effective treatment can demonstrate cost effusiveness in case management.

Following economic changes are seen in producing impact on nursing health care:

- ✓ Supply
- ✓ Demand
- ✓ Policy mechanism
- ✓ Nursing labour market demand and supplies
- ✓ Salary determination
- ✓ Economic back up for nursing practice
- ✓ Health care reimbursement
- ✓ Cost benefit.

Economic issues are challenging current vision of human care. Economics on hospital nurse environment is continuously changing. Interrelationship between economics and nursing can be depicted as under:

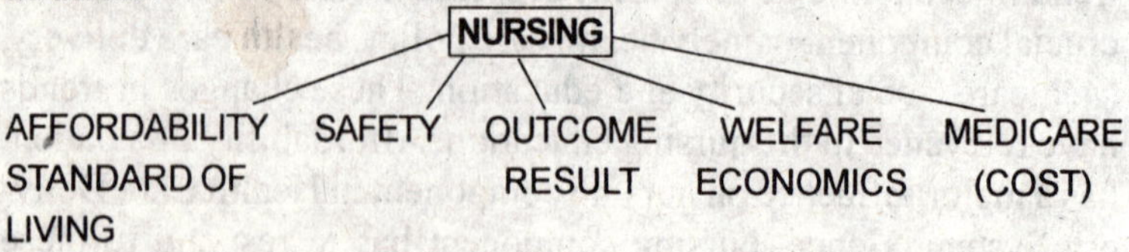

Figure 5.2: Economics and Nursing

Cultural and Social Issues

The issue is the outcome of overpopulation, increased life span and government identification of minority groups in the society that has an influence in nursing education and nursing practice in developing countries like India.

Existing unemployment problem, poverty in society, line of demarcation of below poverty line, low standard of living due to increasing inflation and limited health insurance do influence the nursing education and nursing practice in the country.

Issues in Developed and Developing Countries

Table 5.1: Issues in developed and developing countries

Developed countries (USA, UK, Canada)
Minority proportion is 12 to 14 % Diversity is present in workplace Attitude in contemporary nursing is with hate, contempt, tolerance, respect and celebrations Distribution of 72% whites, 11 percent blacks, remaining others Either student entering or degree holders are about 91% females in the community Student and degree holders among men is about 8 to 9%
Developing countries (India, Pakistan, Sri Lanka)
Minority proportion is 4 to 6 percent Diversity in workplace not significant Attitude in contemporary nursing is with depression (due to unmet basic need) Ignorant, pessimistic, fate determined ideas Distribution is accorded with general, economically backward, and SC and ST Student entering and degree holders are females and are almost 99.9% Among men is insignificant and abut 0.1 percent

6

Sociology for Nurses

The word Sociology was coined by French author Auguste Comte (1798-1857) from his original word social physics. His law was that human efforts to understand world always passes through theological, metaphysical and positive stages. In colloquial words they are termed as supernatural stage, natural stage and scientific stage.

He defined sociology as:
"the investigation of the laws of action and reaction of different parts of social system or social institutions and analysis of society as a unit for progress, change and development".

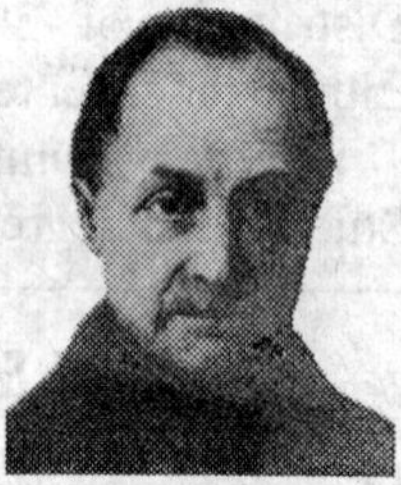

Auguste Comte

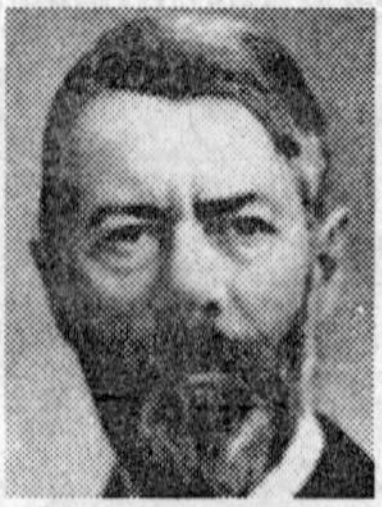

Max Weber

Emile Durkheim defined sociology as:
"the study of social facts"
Karl Mark points out that:
"Sociology deals with social changes primarily by economic influences".

Max Weber (1864-1920) points out:
"the study of organisation of social and economic life according to the principles of efficiency and on the basis of technical knowledge".

This broader definition of sociology includes four elements viz.:
- Social institutions
- Interaction between these institutions
- Society as a unit of study
- Social acts and social relationships.

Complexity of subject matter makes it hard to understand the nature of sociology. There are many social institutions, which are related to each other in different ways giving room for social system. How we live and interact in a society is depicted in sociology. Functioning of family, school, industry, hospital, nursing home, health centre are areas forming part of the study of the nature of sociology.

Wide scope exists in understanding sociology. In a hospital nurse-doctor relationship, nurse-patient relationships, which have common and distinctive features, are found to build up as *social act.*

Nursing sociology in the field of sociology has an area of interest for the study of health disease, health behavior and social medical interactions. We have many social diseases like tuberculosis, leprosy, and sexually transmitted diseases, AIDS though known biological agent causes them. We are turning our interests to study social, behavioral and cultural factors in disease occurrence. Nurse needs to appraise of both biological and behavioral causation of well-being or ill being in human beings.

Historical Milestones:

1832	Study on health of workers. Expressed testing of workers - James Phillip
1838	Social Hygiene – by J A Rochoux
1848	Expressed Term Social Medicine - by Jules Guerin
1848-50	Social Revolution Salomon Neumann Rudolf Virchow Rudolf Leubusher
1902	Term Medical Sociology by E. Blackwell
1910	Book on Medical Sociology by James Warbatte

1911	Theory of Social disease by Grot John
1912	Social Medicine Association developed by Rene Sand.
1925	Social Science by Francis Lee Dunhunn
1933	Study on Environment and health by Edgar Sydenstriker
1943	Institute of Social Medicine at Oxford
1943	John A Ryle- first professor of Social Medicine
1945	F A E Crew - Professor of Social Medicine Edinburgh
1947	Academy of Medicine at New York
1950	René Sand contributions
Late Fifties	Development of sub specialties or Field of Social Medicine Medical Sociology Hospital Sociology Criminal Sociology Demographic Sociology Urban Sociology Rural Sociology Industrial Sociology Religion Sociology Educational Sociology

IMPORTANCE

From the point of view of nursing profession, one has to understand social aspect of disease, how certain predisposing and perpetuating factors influence, how to make nursing profession understandable, acceptable and even affordable by the community. Sociology can help to improve health service facility through:

- Awareness of cultural differences
- Assessment of effects by national policies
- Can lead to self enlightenment or increased self understanding.

His social environment determines health or disease in man. Social and structural factors have direct bearing on the nature of illness; social problems like poverty, poor sanitation and illiteracy influence man on his positive health. A patient either in a hospital or at home has his own habits, customs and beliefs. This new outlook has brought a closer link to man and society.

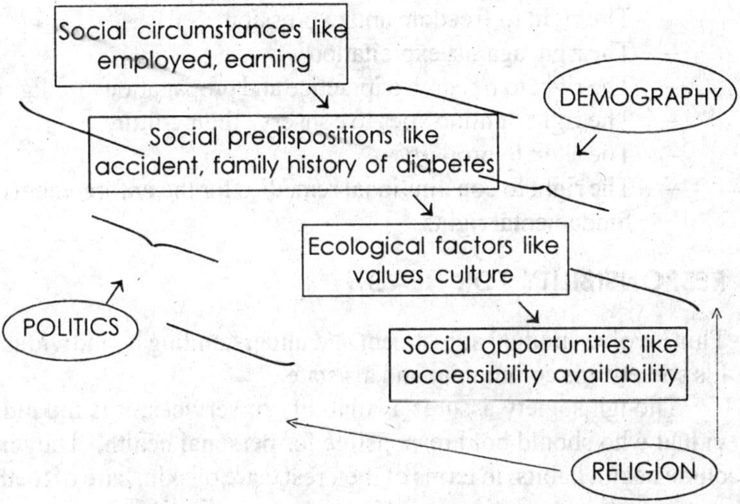

Figure 6.1: Influencing factors in nursing activities

NURSE AS AN INDIVIDUAL

WHO has expressed that "the enjoyment of the highest attainable standard of health is one of the fundamental rights of every human being without distinction of race, religion, political belief, economic or social condition". All countries including India have accepted the above definition and the right to health.

Universal declaration of human rights under article 30 consists:

" All human beings are born free and equal in dignity and rights... everyone has the right to a standard of living adequate for the health and well being of himself and his family, including food, clothing, housing, medical care, necessary social services, right to security in the event of unemployment, sickness, disability, widowhood, old age or other lack of livelihood in circumstances beyond his control .... motherhood and childhood are entitled to special care and assistance. All children born in or out of wedlock shall enjoy the same social protection".

Constitution of India has given guarantee of fundamental rights of individual:

- The right to equality
- The right to freedom and expression
- The right against exploitation
- The right to freedom of practice and propagation of religion
- The right of minorities to conserve their culture
- The right to property
- The right to constitutional remedies for the enforcement of fundamental rights.

RESPONSIBILITY FOR HEALTH

This involves mutual adjustment and understanding by individual, his society, his community and his state.

Though society assures availability of services, it is the individual who should hold responsible for personal health. They include health habits, in terms of diet, rest, care of skin, care of teeth, immunisation, reporting of sick and service utilisation.

SOCIETY

Man has always lived in groups, which is partially or fully organised, and this we call as society. Man cannot live without society. It maintains a standard or laid down principles. Every individual maintain a social relationship, which regulates the human behavior. Here we notice social regulation, law and customs. Effort of an individual is either motivated or is hindered by social norms, which stipulate either right or wrong.

Advancement of Science and Technology as well as Professional activities are either accepted or sometimes not accepted by the society. Thus morbidity, mortality and achievements are directly related to social system, which regulates social relationships.

Structure of Society

There is no satisfactory classification of the society by occupation.

In developed countries classifications like skilled workers, unskilled workers, professionals, labourers etc., are adopted which does not provide uniformity in classification.

Income is used as an economic factor to classify the society into high-income group, middle income and low-income group based on criteria of income earned by an individual. High social class, which seems to enjoy better standard of life have higher incidence of metabolic disorders and higher incidence of psychosomatic disorders.

Caste system predominates in developing countries especially in India. Society was basically classified by the caste system into four main divisions viz., – *Brahmin, Kshatriyas, Vaishyas and Shudras*. They are further subdivided into sub castes. Social rules and social regulations relating to rituals, marriages and food are seen.

Characteristics of Society

Table 6.1: Characteristics of society

Tribal	Agricultural	Industrial
Hunting era Close net society Faster cultural belief Faster religious belief Ceremony, Myth, Magic predominate	Cultivation era Animal rearing for food Traditional family Mores, Folkway predominate	Revolution era No traditional families Drug abuse present Sex trade present Anti social activities present

Urban Society and Rural Society

Indian society is mainly rural in nature, which constitutes 78% of population. There are about 7 lakh villages and each village is with a population of 500 to 2000. Villages are self-sufficient. They are mainly agrarian in nature where agriculture is taken up as the main livelihood.

Large, dense and permanent settlement form urban area, which form 22% of population. According to 2001 census there are 8637 towns and cities. Now there are 300 mega cities indicating extent of urbanisation. We come across occupational diversity and impersonal social life.

There is wide difference between urban and rural society in terms of health aspect, like disease pattern, socioeconomic characteristics, demography, and availability of health manpower, health status and nature of health problem.

The major differences between urban and rural society are depicted in Table 6.2.

Table 6.2: Difference between urban and rural society

	Rural society	Urban society
Disease pattern	Infections	Metabolic diseases and cancer diseases
Socioeconomic characteristics	Rural Joint family Agriculture occupation Low per capita income Low literacy rate Low standard of living Poor medical care	Urban Single family Industry occupation High per capita income High literacy rate High standard of living Good medical care
Demography	More young population Paediatric problems High birth rate High death rate High growth rate High IMR High MMR Low life expectancy	More older population Geriatric problems Low birth rate Low death rate Low growth rate Low IMR Low MMR High life expectancy
Health problems	Infection and malnutrition	Obesity, Non communicable diseases
Health manpower	Shortage	More than adequate

Social Mobility

Indian society is a *closed class* system. There is restricted movement of social ladder. People changing their religion, caste and race are not commonly found. Recently urbanisation and civilisation is making people accept social mobility on the basis of gaining wealth or on the basis of achievement.

Nature of Society as Biosocial System

Biosocial system of society is made up of values, customs, tradition and conventions. This system keeps a standardised ways of action to survive longer and face time tested odd situations. Natural calamities, man made conflicts have made this biosocial system to survive their test of time. Each biosocial system will have varied social system like primitive, civilised and moderately rigid in terms of sociological manifestations. A society can be with well advanced science and technology and show open class societies mainly thriving for achievement and progress. Biosocial system of society is influenced by:

- Civil unrest
- Social problems including crime
- Unemployment
- Overgrowth of population.

Evolution of Society

Literacy, standard of living and population movement determines evolution of society.

Urbanisation and civilisation are bringing revolutionary changes in a society where we see over-density of population and a shift from primary occupation to secondary and tertiary occupation.

Special type of urbanisation has developed called metropolitanisation where central city shows economic dominance over surrounding cities.

This evolutionary change brings following changes in a society. They are:

- Demographic changes
- Ecological changes
- Behavioural changes
- Health changes.

Social System

Social system enrolls individual, family, community and society at large. It provokes many social institutions. Social system is seen, as Weber puts it, "in all human behavior insofar as the acting individual attach subjective meaning to it".

Society differs from each other; they simulate each other in a social system.

The system has identifiable institutions like family, school, college, hospital, nursing homes, industry and the like. Thus it deals with societies and institutions.

Various identified social relationships are manifolds of social system, structure, function and mechanism of social system.

Society in a social system has its structure and stratification. They can be described as under:

Social structure (Social anatomy)

- Socioeconomic groups like upper, upper middle, middle, lower middle, lower
- Professional groups like doctors, nurses, engineers
- Religious groups like Hindu, Muslim, Christian
- Caste groups like four major group with subgroups among Hindus
- Demographic groups like young, old, male, female
- Geographic or area groups like rural suburban urban suburban.

Social function (Social physiology)

This explains ventilation (respiration), nutrition (gastrointestinal), waste disposal (excretion), removal of offenders in the society (vital organ) depicted as manifold functions of the society.

Social problems (Social pathology)

It describes pathology of society like infant deaths, protein energy malnutrition etc., in the social system.

Sociological problems detection (Social diagnosis)

Survey, screening and surveillance help us to identify social pathology and risk factors in health and disease.

Social management (Social therapy)

Personal or group health education, counselling, social welfare activities, social security measures form social therapy in social system.

Role

In social system we have many roles to play like son, daughter, brother, sister, teacher, lecturer, priest, mother, father, grandfather, grandmother and the like. These role plays demarcate our relationships within a social system. Role confirms the behavior of an individual to differentiate with others in the group. When it is given by virtue of age sex etc., it is called *ascribed role*. By virtue of education and experience when done it is *achieved role*. We play our role as nurses and doctors in health care services. When training is given to a nurse it is called **Role Induction.**

Status

Status is an achieved role in the community or society. It can be head of the family, head of the state and head of the country. This is possible by social selection and is demarcated with political activities. Status gives power to produce or to modify norms, values and customs. It is also called a social honour or prestige accorded to a person by society. Such status groups follow their own life style and behavior pattern. According to a sociologist status may be positive or negative. Group leader is a positive status and outcast is negative status.

Race

On the basis of biologically grouped features, many competencies are assigned to a group or to individuals who demonstrate a set of social relationships. Many attributes of biological origin help to differentiate a group, which is called race.

Social Interaction and Social Process

Social interaction includes both formal and informal situations in which people meet one another. In nursing profession interaction between tutor and a nurse is formal social interaction. The same tutor and nurse when meet in a class social it becomes social interaction of informal type.

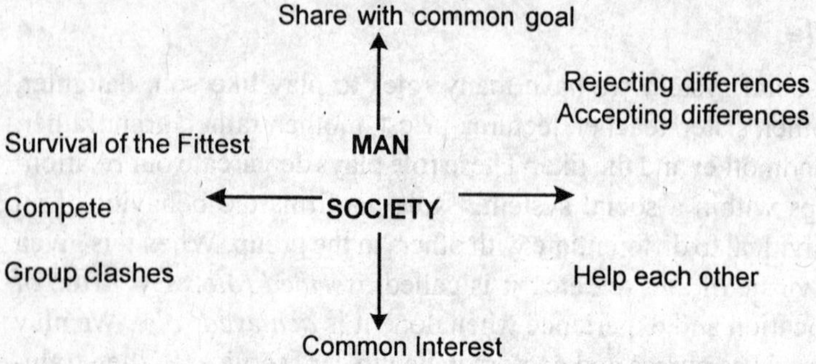

Figure 6.2: Social interactions

Social interaction includes both formal and informal situations in which people meet one another. In nursing profession interaction between tutor and a nurse is formal social interaction. The same tutor and nurse when meet in a class social it becomes social interaction of informal typc.

Social process is a long-term effective behavior-moulding step, which involve many formal and informal interactions. Child developing social norm and values at home with mother is a social process, which is termed as *socialization.*

A positive outlook in social interaction and social process is seen with cooperation, completion, accommodation and assimilation. In assimilation values and norms of a dominant culture is taken up by a week group in a society. During social process an acceptance of minority group by a majority group is through acceptance of norms of majority.

A negative outlook in social interaction is seen with conflict and isolation. A non interactive individual or a group is said to be isolated in the social process. Conflict is a sociological perspective of competition. When a group struggles to gain access to and to control resources, conflict is seen as a social process, which allow tension and divisions.

Socialisation

It is a social process where man inducts his role as an individual in a family, society or community. He gains the knowledge of norms, values, sanctions and customs in the process of socialisation.

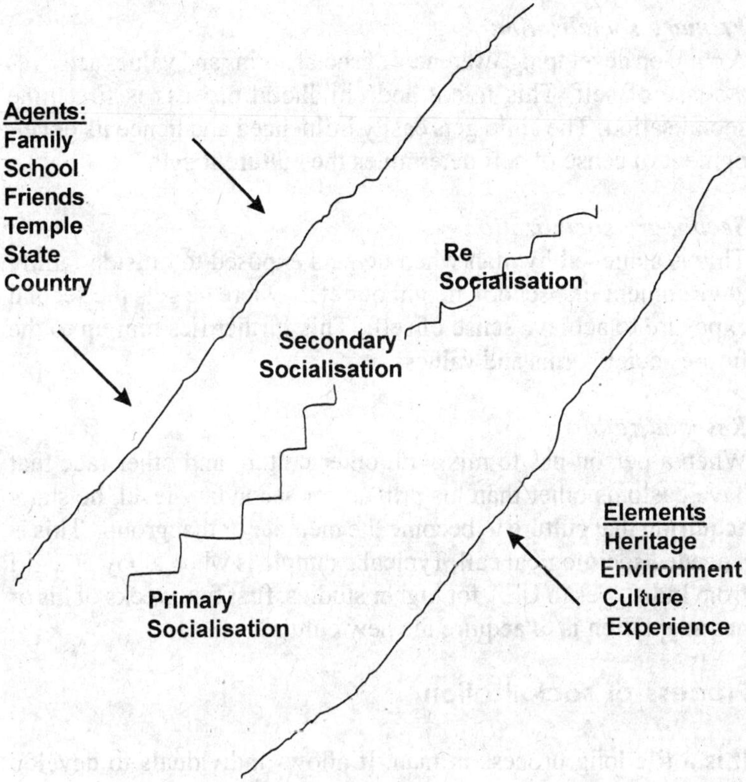

Figure 6.3: Steps to socialization

Co-related Terminologies in Social Medicine

Socialised Medicine:

This is a type of health care by the nation wherein free and subsidized medical care is given to all citizens.

Group Dynamics:

This sphere of social medicine studies the response of the community to illness particularly for social diseases and what a community adopts measures for self help. It deals with group reactions and group responses.

Primary socialization

A child on developing awareness of social norms and values achieves a sense of self. This infant and childhood process is first time socialisation. The child gets easily influenced and hence its development of sense of self determines the culture it gets.

Secondary socialization

This is achieved by man when he gets exposed to outside family environment like school, neighbour etc., where he gets the second exposure to achieve sense of self. This further ties him up to the future social norms and values.

Resocialization

When a person has to mix with other culture and other race that have customs other than his primary or secondary level, he starts acquiring that culture to become the member of that group. This is a needed sociological call. Typical example is when a boy or a girl from India goes to USA for higher studies, first few weeks of his or her adaptation is to acquire the new culture.

Process of socialization

It is a life long process in man. It allows individuals to develop themselves and their potential, to learn and to make adjustments.

Freud has postulated that dependency, fear, need for sympathy and love takes the child to social process of socialisation where he or she may replicate the values and culture of parents and other relatives.

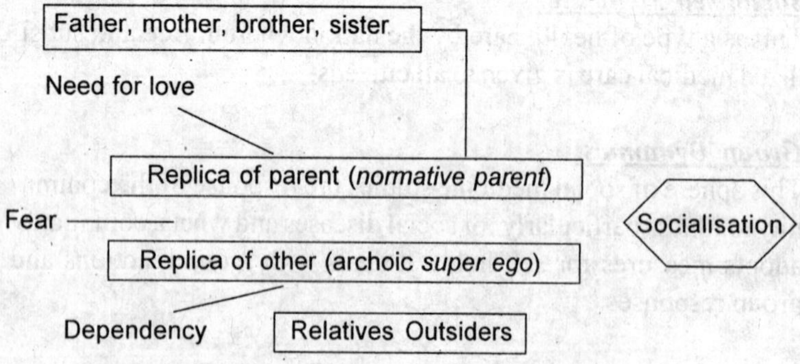

Figure 6.4: Socialisation model after Freud

Principles of socialisation is used in nursing training where we do *role induction*. During nursing profession, set of norms are achieved by the nurse in this condition.

Self Importance of Socialisation and Individualisation

Person undergoes transformation through imitation and identification. This can be within the family, which is called normative parent, or outside the family, which is called *archaic super ego*. This has great relevance in making a person as required good member of a society. Blending and fusion of personalities are looked upon with great care for personality development and for individualisation.

Social control

Human social behaviour is regulated by many factors. At family level we come across social regulations and in a society we see law and enactment. These are to regulate social behaviour towards normal and have the control over deviation from normal.

Rewards and *punishments* control behaviour. Standardised social interactions become *customs*. Among them a few are stringent and are called *mores*. They become *social regulations* when we make them as formal one. Cultural standards in a society are termed as value orientation. *Fashion* is a typical example of valuc orientation in social control. Right way of doing things in society is called *folkway*. Most of the occasions, folkways are done by reflex and do not carry vital importance.

In nursing profession we have many social controls for an effective nursing career. Code of conduct and dress code is a formal social control enforced in nursing profession. Similarly nurses take an oath in oath taking ceremony, which can be regarded as informal social control of the institution.

Social group

Any number of individuals when interact or when perceive creating a sense of WE, or THEY, then a social group is formed. There are many uses of a social group. They are to solve a problem, to reduce anxiety and tension, to attain a goal and to have cooperation. Types of human groups are:

- Primary group
- Secondary group
- In group
- Out group
- Economic group
- Political group
- Religious group.

Members of a particular social group feel committed to conduct themselves for a required expectation. Various theories are postulated in social group formation. They are:

- Human wants nearness (Proximity)
- Cooperation to achieve goals (George Homan Theory)
- Sharing commonness (New Comb Theory)
- Mutual comparison and reward (Theory of Tibut and Kelly).

A social group can be small or big. It can be a temporary or permanent by nature.

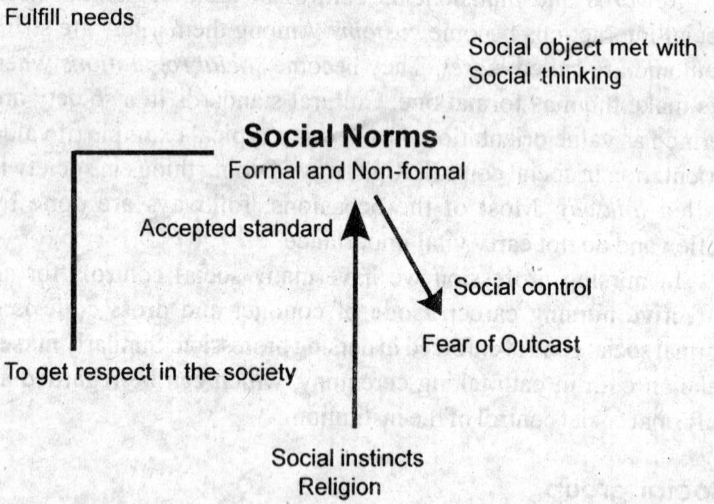

Figure 6.5: Social norms

Crowd, Public and Audience

These are temporary without any commonness. They are just an emotional group and do not have goal oriented activities. Colloquially it is called MOB and mob mentality is described as a gathering when there is no need, when one cannot perceive any reason or when one cannot interact in a group.

COMMUNITY

World Health Organisation has defined community as "group of individuals and families living together in a defined geographic area, usually comprising of a village, a town, or a city". The community usually has shown common interest, which has some common characteristic features. They are:

- Live in a defined geographic area
- People live together with certain social regulations
- They show cooperative effort in day to day life
- They establish requisite sub organisations like hospital, bank, store, school, college, market and industry.

Human network is found established in a given community. At a given point of time we see all categories of people with different spectrum from health point of view. At a given point of time we also find healthy group, apparently healthy group, sick but ambulatory group, sick hospitalised group, chronically sick, dying and dead. Communities have varied economic functions. Directly or indirectly they are grouped on the basis of their occupation for the purpose of categorisation. They are:

1. Primary occupation like agriculture, forestry, fishing, mining
2. Secondary occupation like manufacturing, processing, fabricating, auto industry
3. Tertiary occupations like education, health service, recreation etc.

Present Grouping of Community

a. *Rural community:* Villages form a specified boundary, specified independent occupation and specified administrative set up.

b. *Standard urban area:* A town with a population of 50,000 having encroachment of rural community with mutual socioeconomic link.

c. *Urban agglomeration:* A few cities with good growth with delineated boundary.

d. *Urban community:* Population density is seen more than 400 person per square kilometer and is declared urban area by government.

e. *Cosmopolitan community:* Mega cities with above 3 lakh population, specified geographic boundary and defined under city municipal corporations.

Difference Between Society and Community

Society is a group of people who settle down permanently and organise themselves. This shows a social system with demonstrable social relationships between individuals. Here behaviors of individual are regulated by social regulations. Society changes from time to time as a dynamic process. It incorporates one or more community.

Community is a social group determined by a markable boundary. It shows common values and common interest. It demarcates a geographical area to map out a village, a town, a city or a nation. Community is a network of human relationships. Community is a major functioning unit of society; our house is located in a community; our children are educated in a community. Human basic needs are met with in the community.

FAMILY

Definition

" It is a group of individuals who are biologically related and live together and eat from a common kitchen."

They share House and social environment and hence a family is called a **social unit** or a **cultural unit.**

By removing the word biologically related, the unit becomes a HOUSEHOLD.

Types of family

a) Nuclear family: This is an elementary family of married couple and their children, who live together in the same household.

Social characteristics of nuclear family:

Urban based
Industralised areas
Western culture amalgamated
Change of life style is accepted
Independent and unstable families
Female empowerment exists
Low values for religious and cultural values
It has weaknesses

b) Joint family: This has more than one married couple and their children, who live together in the same household.

Social characteristics of joint family:

Division of labour is present
Get leisure time
Give importance to social values
Lacks sustained effort for existence
Dependency present
Privacy and individuality is little
Litigations and clashes among members present
Parenthood partial

c) Three generation family: When married son or daughter live with their parents along with their children.

d) Extended family: When old generation live, unmarried children live, polyandrous and polygamous couple live, married daughters live in father's house (matrilocal), married sons live in in-law's house (patrilocal), extended family is formed.

Family Cycle

There are four stages:

Stage 1 : Stage of formation when couple marry

Stage 2 : Stage of growth when children are born

Stage 3 : Stage of retraction when children marry and go away

Stage 4 : Stage of disintegration when death of one or both parent occur.

Functions of The Family

1. Childbirth and child rearing
2. Sexual gratification
3. Primary socialisation of individual occurs
4. Social and mental stress are overcome
5. Social and economic support is obtained
6. Social interaction brings about new knowledge
7. Each member has a role play and a job responsibility.

Family Problem

1. Infertility, sterility
2. Adaptation
3. Egoism
4. Marital disharmony
5. Broken family
6. Poor social interaction
7. Divorce
8. Economic problem
9. Malnutrition
10. Alcoholism
11. Conflict due to non adaptation of culture
12. Susceptibility to diseases
13. Chronic illness in the family.

Marriage

Marriage is socially approved social relations, which allow sexual relationship between two individuals of opposite sex. Marriage form basis of a family of procreation with an expectation that married couple will produce and bring up children.

Deviant marriage

Modern families are seen with homosexual marriages, which do not serve the purpose of marriage. Similarly polygamy or polyandry is deviant marriages, which form extended families as seen in certain religions.

Modern families

Pattern of family is getting changed due to accessibility and availability of social and economic sanctions. When both couple are earning members child rearing is by a contract worker. Marriage is not a permanent bond and the Act of Divorce legally permits leaving to separate and live to separate. Following outcomes are seen in modern families:

- Lone parent household
- Remarriages
- Female partner to head the family
- Violence and abuse in the family
- Low accordance to family values.

Change in Indian family

Slowly size of the family, type of the family and composition of the family are changing due to varied social interactions and progressive urbanisation and civilisation. Slowly there has been reduction in joint family or three generation family. Average size of family has come down from 6.3 to 3.1.

This change has lead to loosening social regulation, lacking role of family in health and disease. Indian women, like western culture, face difficulty in reproductive and child health period, which used to be taken care of by elderly women at home. Kinship in the family is slowly deteriorating. Nuclear family is predominant mainly because of industrialisation of societies. Divorce rate is increasing giving room for reduced number of first marriages. Thus there is considerable diversity in family norms.

Legislation on Indian marriage and family

Family law, Hindu law cover the legal implications of divorce, remarriage, property dispute and care taken towards offspring which regulate the social problem from time to time.

As a policy measure age at marriage for a boy and girl have been fixed at 18 and 21 years respectively. This dictum is given as a family welfare planning measure.

Civil marriage and registered marriage are allowed as per Marriage Act in India. As per Registration of Births, Deaths and Marriage Act, registration of marriage (even after civil marriage) is made mandatory.

Since social regulation is not found useful in social control over family issues, legislation on Indian marriage is put into action for allowing smooth and effective family pattern.

The urban families

Since population is getting concentrated in urban areas due to industrialisation with varied occupation, urban family has moulded to a pattern, which need consideration in a social system. This has lead to urban crisis, which is a direct impact of increased exponential urban growth (now it is 3.09%).

Urban families are facing following economic, social and health problems:

Health problems:	Diarrhoea, STD, hepatitis, skin infection, malignancy
Social problems:	Alcoholism, drug abuse, prostitution
Environmental problems:	Road accidents, atmosphere pollution (air pollution, water pollution, soil pollution)
Economic problems:	Poverty
Psychological problems:	Stress, anxiety, neurosis, suicide

Family problems enumerated above are mainly due to both poverty and prosperity and hence are called:

a) **Poverty induced** and

b) **Prosperity induced** family problems.

Healthy family movement is determined by social interactions and civic amenities like

- Small family norm
- Quality and quantity of food
- Healthy environment
- Slum improvement measures.

Urban and rural contrast with respect to family can be tabulated as under (Table 6.3):

Table 6.3: Urban and rural contrast for family

Item	Rural	Urban
Population	Thin	Dense
Occupation	Agriculture	Varied
Social dependance	Social reliant	Dependent
Social interaction	Primary	Secondary
Caste system	Dominant	Not dominant
Geographic boundary	Small	Big
Residential area	Not planned	Planned

Social Stratification

Social inequality is present in all types of communities. In some it may be by race while in others it may be by caste.

Ranking of social activities according to values are age old phenomena. This is a requirement for functioning of society. Another cause of social classification seems to hold position and power in a society.

Health implications:

a) Social class is related to certain types of diseases. Malnutrition among low socioeconomic class, hypertension among high socioeconomic class illustrates the relation

b) Susceptibly or risk group identification is possible

c) Health service planning is possible

Social Classification

By occupation: We come across this classification in Britain (Registrar General of England) (Table 6.4).

Table 6.4: Socioeconomic class by occupation

Social class	Occupation
I	Professional
II	Managerial
III	Skilled
IV	Semiskilled
V	Unskilled

By education: Illiterate, literate, primary, secondary, metric, graduation, post graduation are noted grouping for social classification

Awareness, knowledge, practice with respect to health programme and disease are related to educational status.

By Pareek method: For rural areas, Pareek has evolved a method by considering caste, occupation, education, social participation, land holding, housing, farm power, material possession and type of family. It is a form of scoring system for social stratification.

By income: Income alone is not considered for social classification. It gives value of socioeconomic grouping. However with other variables, many methods are adopted in research methodology.

Prasad Classification (updated By income in Rupees)

Social class	Prasad 1961	Updated (1) 1991	Updated (2) 2001	Updated (3) 2009 (March) (Rounded off to hundreds)
I	100 & above	1021 & above	20503 & above	19555 &above
II	50-99	510-1020	10230-20499	9800-19554
III	30-49	306-509	6130-10229	5900-9799
IV	15-29	154-305	3076-6129	2950-5899
V	Below 15	Below 153	Below 3075	Below 2949

1991 inflation index = 206, consumer index = 4.96

$$\text{Correction factor} = \frac{206 \times 4.96}{100} = 10.2176$$

2001 inflation index = 406, consumer index = 5.05

$$\text{Correction factor} = \frac{406 \times 5.05}{100} = 20.503$$

2006 inflation index = 480, consumer index = 5.45

$$\text{Correction factor} = \frac{480 \times 5.45}{100} = 26.160$$

2009 March inflation index = 582, consumer index = 3.36

Correction Factor = 19.555

$$\text{Correction factor} = \frac{\text{(cost inflation index) x (current price index)}}{100}$$

Note: C.F. (correction factor) is calculated based on Cost Inflation Index (COI) and Current Price Index for the year 1991, 2001 and 2009 March are considered.

As per calculation **100 of 1961 is equal to 1021 at 1991,**
1000 of 1991 is equal to 20503 at 2001,
1000 of 2001 is equal to 26160 at 2006,
1000 of 2006 is equal to 19555 at 2009 March.

$$\text{Correction Factor} = \frac{\text{(cost inflation index)} \times \text{(current price index)}}{100}$$

As per calculation 100.00 of 1961 is equal to 1021 at 1991, 20503 at 2001, 29900 at 2004 and 19555 at 2009 March.

Note: Estimates are done by the author for teaching purpose and the source is from Reserve Bank of India, The Economic Times, I I M Lucknow and National dailies (March 2009 data).

Kuppuswamy Classification (Modified)

	Item			Score
A.	Education	Professional, PG		7
		Graduate		6
		Inter		5
		High school		4
		Middle school		3
		Primary		2
		Illiterate		1
B.	Occupation	Profession		10
		Semiprofession		6
		Clerk, shop, farm		5
		Skilled		4
		Semi skilled		3
		Unskilled		2
		Unemployed		1
C.	Income (per capita)	800 and above*	(16000-11999)@	12
		400-799	(12000-9999)	10
		300-399	(10000-7999)	6
		200-299	(8000-5999)	4
		120-199	(6000-3999)	3
		40-199	(4000-3999)	2
		below 40	(below 2000)	1

* as per 88-89 index

@ Figure in parenthesis are as per 2008-09 indexTotal score = A + B + C

Social class	Score (total)	as per 2008-09 index
I	26-29	(16000 and above)
II	16-25	(10000-15999)
III	11-15	(5000-9999)
IV	5-10	(2000-4999)
V	Below 5	(Below 2000)

Prabhakara Classification*

Classification of belonging and achievement 1982

	Score			
	0	*1*	*2*	*3*
House	Rented	Lease	Own	—
Room	Nil	1-2	3+	—
Toilet	Shared	Separate	—	—
Kitchen	Not separate	Separate	—	—
Vehicle	Nil	Two wheeler (mechanised)	Two wheeler (auto driven)	—
Radio/Tape recorder	Nil	Own one	Own two	—
Father's Education	Illiterate	Primary	Secondary/ technical	University
Number of living children	7	3-6	1-2	—

Social class:

I	0-3
II	4-6
III	7-9
IV	10-12
V	13-15

Pareek classification for rural areas

This is based on the following characteristics

1. Caste
2. Occupation of head of the family
3. Education of head of the family
4. Social participation level
5. land holding by the head
6. Farm power in terms of bullocks, tractors, ox, sheep, horse
7. Housing
8. Material possession
9. Family type.

Socio economic scoring by grades

Caste	
OC	10
BC	8
SC	6
Occupation	
Professional	10
Semiprofessional	6
Clerks, shops keepers	5
Skilled worker	4
Semiskilled worker	3
Unskilled worker	2
Not employed	1
Literacy	
PG	7
UG	6
Inter	5
Metric	4
Middle school	3
Primary school	2
Illiterate	1
Literacy of housewife	
Degree	8
Inter	7
Metric	6
Primary	6
Illiterate	1
Type of family	
Nuclear	6
Joint	4

Housing		
Own		6
Rented		2
House type		
Pucca		10
Semipucca		6
Kutcha		3
Land holding		
Dry land 30 acres/wet land 15 acres		10
20-30 acres/10-15 acres		8
10-20 acres/5-10 acres		6
5-10 acres/2-3 acres		4
Below 5 acres/below 2 acres		3
No land/no land		1
Farm power		
Tractor		12
Bullock/ ox		2 each
Horse , cow, buffalo		3 each
Donkey		1 each
Sheep or goat		½ each
Material possession		
A C		12
Colour TV		8
Air cooler		6
Fridge		6
B/W TV		4
Fans		2 each
Social participation		
Good		6
Rare		3
Nil		1

Total score

90	Upper class
75-90	Higher middle
60-75	Middle
45-60	Lower middle
30-45	Lower classes
below 30	Below poverty line (BPL)

By caste: Classification is no longer valid because of its sensitive and intricate nature. In India people do not easily change their caste or religion. It is called CLOSED CLASS. Movement of the social ladder by caste or religion is restricted and has influenced progressive movement. The movement in social ladder is called SOCIAL MOBILITY, which brings about transformation. Social transformation of people is met with social resistance.

Presently in India social classification like upper caste, other caste, scheduled caste, scheduled tribe, other backward caste are in use for social welfare activities.

Wealth Index

This is defined as an index of the economic status of households. This reflects health service and health outcome. Major determinants are household income, health services and health outcome. Characteristics that are considered under this are:

- Household electrification
- Window type
- Source of drinking water
- Toilet facility
- Flooring
- Exterior mosaic
- Roof
- Cooking gas
- Ownership
- Overcrowding
- Ownership of bank account, belongings including vehicle

Urban wealth index = 48% and rural is 7%.

This index is inversely proportional to Infant Mortality Rate in the community.

Human Poverty Index

This is introduced in 1997. It describes average achievements in human basic needs.

Human Poverty Index = $\{[\ 1/3\ P_1^{\alpha} + P_2^{\alpha} + P_3^{\alpha}\ ]\}^{1/\alpha}$

Where

P1 = probability at birth of not surviving to age 40 which is 17.0 at present

P2 = adult literacy rate which is 40% now

P3 = unweighted average of proportion not using potable water and

Children under weight for age, which is 30 at present

$\alpha = 3$

Current data : Not using potable water= 15%

Children underweight for age = 48%

By above data Human Poverty Index = $\{[1/3\ 17^3 + 40^3 + 30^3]\}^{1/3}$
= 30%

Rural Community in India

About 71 percent of population live in rural community in over 700,000 villages. Government of India has three tier system of health care for primary health care through village health guide, anganwadi worker and traditional birth attendant.

Health profile of villages:

a. Health problems	Infection, malnutrition, poor sanitation, shortage of health personnel
b. Demographic picture	More young people with paediatric problem, high rates of birth, death, growth, infant mortality, Maternal mortality and low life expectation
c. Socioeconomic picture	Joint family system with agriculture as occupation, low rates of per capita income, literacy rate, standard of living and medical care

Change in Indian rural life: A Panchayat raj system has come into effect to uplift villages and for democratic decentralisation. Three tier system of local self government is as under:

Gram Panchayat	–	at village level
Mandal Panchayat	–	at block level
Zilla Parishad	–	at district level

Gram panchayat is responsible for village improvement. Cooperative movement has brought cooperatives in agriculture, bank, marketing to facilitate village upliftment.

Following Government of India programmes are approved from time to time for Rural development and for social and economic growth. They are:

1. Indira Awaz Yojana—*shelter to the shelterless*
2. Jawahar Rozgar Yojana (JRY)—*sustained employment*
3. Employment Assurance Scheme (EAS)—*assured employment*
4. Million Wells Scheme (MWS)—*open irrigation wells*
5. Integrated Rural Development Programme (IRDP)
6. Development of Women and Children in Rural Areas (DWACRA)
7. Training of Rural Youth for Self Employment (TRYSEM)
8. Supply of Toolkits to Rural Artisans
9. Land Reforms (surplus land distribution)
10. Waste land development
11. Old age pension scheme
12. Rural Women Delivery Allowance.

Culture

Definitions

Culture is an accumulation of thoughts, values and objects; it is a social heritage acquired by us from preceding generations through leasing as distinguished from the biological heritage which is passed on to us automatically through genes. (Graham Wall).

Folkway is the recognized or accepted ways of behaviour in society (MacIver).

Mores is best reserved for those customs, which are fairly strong feelings of the rightness or wrongness of modes of behaviour (Edward Sapir).

Culture is defined as values, ceremonies and ways of life characteristic of a given social group. Culture is one of the most distinctive properties of human social association. Culture stands for mode of living, language, custom and belief. Hence it is socially acquired and learned behaviour.

Cultural diversity is seen with diversity of human behaviour and his practice. Small and big societies have monoculture and multicultural practice respectively. Sub culture refers to a segment of population showing a change in cultural pattern.

Cultural pattern in India (some examples):

Health and disease	– it is by supernatural factor
	– it is by sin of past life
Personal hygiene	– bathing everyday done
	– apply oil before bath
	– pan, supari, lime eaten as custom
	– hukka smoking is a custom
	– walking barefoot common
Environmental hygiene	– open field defaecation
	– washing of cloth, washing of animal and ablution at pond
RCH	– certain foods are avoided in pregnancy, lactation and in infancy
	– delivery is conducted by untrained indigenous dai
	– new born is not given colostrum
	– cow dung application to cut end of the umbilical cord
	– skin branding for headache
Nutrition	– higher caste do not eat non vegetarian food
	– certain foods are hot
	– certain foods are cold
	– eating garlic is a taboo

Above illustration gives us the cultural pattern of people which have direct bearing on health activities.

Understanding of culture is important to bring about changes in habit, custom and belief of the community, with respect to health of the individual and the community.

Trans-cultural society

Cultures that influence health are more emphasized in a trans-cultural society. Lung cancer is increasing as the people have accepted smoking habit as culture. Liver cirrhosis is increasing as the people have accepted alcohol habit as culture. Social habits by different cultures are mingled in a society to form trans-cultural society, which speaks of ways of living.

Social Change

It is an alteration in the basic structure of a social group. Social change is continuously occurring social phenomenon in life. They are now intense in modern era. There has been a tremendous shift from traditional system to modern social system.

Following are the determinants of social change:

i. Demographic	:	age, sex, occupation, education
ii. Behaviorur	:	suicide, homicide, delinquency, sexual offense
iii. Culture	:	values, custom
iv. Social structure	:	family pattern, social control
v. Environment	:	physical, political and cultural

Change in social system in modern period is mainly due to economic influence, political influence and cultural influence.

Social change indicators are:

a. Development of science and Technology
b. Agriculture development
c. Modernisation of Industry
d. Ecological changes.

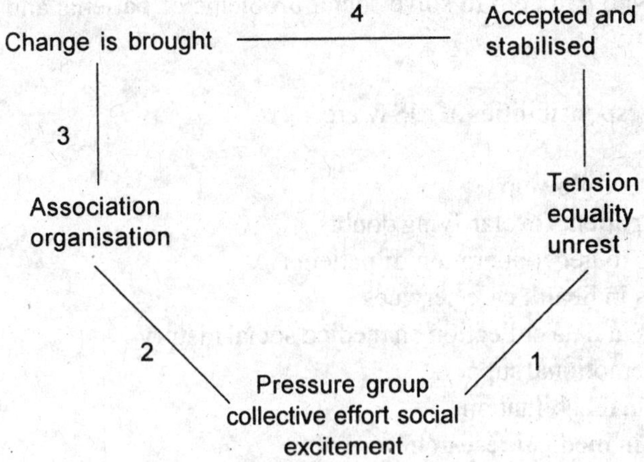

Figure 6.6: Social change cycle

Standard of Living

It refers to ways of living as shown by spending capacity and acquiring capacity. This depends on:

a. National income
b. Total production
c. Population growth
d. Educational level.

Standard of living is related to health and disease. High standard of living brings down diarrhoea, cholera, tuberculosis and it improves standard of health status in population. Standard of living determines birth rate, death rate, nutritional level and life expectancy.

MEDICAL SOCIAL WORKER (MSW)

He is a Postgraduate in Medical social work or Sociology who is initially appointed to the department of Preventive and Social Medicine for the work in their Field Practice Areas namely Urban Health Training Centres and Rural Health Training Centres.

Nowadays they are appointed in mental hospitals, child guidance clinics, cancer hospitals, F.P. clinics, STD clinics and de-addiction centres.

MSW is person who can fill the gap between hospital and community, who can help to solve social problems of patients and of community.

Specific responsibilities of MSW are:

- Help in follow up
- Help patients in clarifying doubts
- Helps to get cooperation of patients
- Helps in health care services
- Helps in data collection on medico social history
- Give emotional support
- Help in rehabilitation
- Help in medical research
- Help in communication activities.

7

Psychology for Nurses

INTRODUCTION

Psychology is concerned with human behavior. Both physical factors and mental factors, which mean bodily action and function as well as mental action and function, interact with each other which is more complicated than a circuit or computer.

Man in his society is influenced by values, attitude, economic conditions, and interaction with other members of his family, his co-workers in his working placement, his religious placement and other social system. Social stratification and gender differences have limited the normal behavior of people.

Man has set certain do's and don'ts in his setting. His Behaviour is determined by these factors. Acceptance or a sanction for treatment is also determined by his Behaviour.

In nursing care we come across following type Behaviour which directs the individual towards acceptance or rejection of care:

Health Behaviour

Oral hygiene, care of teeth, care of genital organs, periodic health check up to identify risks at early phase, eating habit, sleeping habit, bowel habit etc., are examples of health behaviour. They help in prevention of many diseases. Monogamy and marital harmony is another example of health behaviour, which prevents STD and AIDS.

Illness Behaviour

In early part of sickness home remedy from enquiry with friends, advices from elders are common. This is a natural reaction to subjective manifestations of a disease. On the contrary, health awareness helps in early diagnosis and prompt treatment.

Treatment Behaviour

Acceptance or non-acceptance of activities suggested for disease form treatment behaviour. Some like oral drugs, others parenteral (injections) at advice. Many are scared of surgery and go for medical treatment only. In nursing care, taking drugs or medicamentation as directed and return for follow up and advice is regarded as good treatment behaviour.

Definition of psychology

"The study of human behaviour, the study of how people behave, the study of why they behave and which are within accepted norm".

Scope of psychology

Psychology is glued with every aspect of human life. It is seen in all types of human interaction. Understanding of human mind helps us to analyses intricacies involved in mental disorders. There are various branches of psychology, which deal with day-to-day occurrence in human behaviour. These branches are:

1. Social psychology
2. Educational psychology
3. Child psychology
4. Applied psychology
5. Psycho analysis
6. Medical psychology (Psychiatry)

7. Adult psychology
8. Women psychology
9. Elders psychology.

Application of psychology in nursing profession

Psychology helps a nurse in understanding the need of a patient. Nurse can motivate patient for required helpful activity useful for recovery. She can make patient think and reason out in medical emergencies. Understanding emotions and feelings of the sick will be the secret of success in effective nursing care. Psychotherapy may be required in cases of psychosomatic disorders like asthma, peptic ulcer, ulcerative colitis, hypertension etc.,

Methods adopted in psychology as a science of behavior in abnormal behavior and mental illness areas are psychoanalysis, psycho diagnosis, psychosocial counselling and psychotherapy.

Interest

Humans show interest for security, for pleasure and for self esteem. Caste, language, religion and social status also command interest.

Social interest can shape a personality. Social interest by man shapes communication and perception of man.

Human behavior

Human Behavior is human response to his surroundings. When we see a snake we run away; when we see a coin lying on the ground, we go near and pick it up; when a person spit on us we hit that person. Here snake, coin and spitting on the face are stimulus and running away, picking up and hitting are responses. It is an old age dictum that stimulus determines our behaviour.

Response by lower animals is at lower level of function. Man responds at higher order of functioning and he uses integrated and coordinated responses.

Integrated response

Man as higher animal uses integrated and consolidated response as a response to stimulus. Habits and skills are used by reflex. Emotions, feeling and tension are created as automated response. But man uses thinking, reasoning and perceptions, which are intellectual response.

Functioning level of stimuli

Behaviour (conscious)

As per the standards and norms in social system man behaves to external stimuli like touch, smell which are determined by cerebral cortex. Nurse standing and greeting the matron is a reflex process but standardised code of behaviour, which is stimulated by the sight of matron.

Behaviour (subconscious)

These arise within our body and level of functioning is in thalamus of the brain. This response is in terms of emotions and feelings. Anger, joy, sympathy, affection are response from subconscious behavior to natural occurrences. Death, birth and loss of leg by accident are typical examples to produce this behaviour.

Behaviour (unconscious)

Opposite to conscious behavior, man many times, responds to certain stimuli without his knowledge. When a person witnesses "great suffering to die" he is bound to pronounce many things, which did not happen at all. Very bad event in life, which is totally avoided even with stimuli, constitute unconscious behavior.

Behaviour (intellectual)

Thinking, reasoning and analysis of situation before response is a high order functioning. This type is diagnostic to man as a behaving organism.

Attention and Perception

Attention and perception are two major mental activities. Attention is an alternate to observation. They have lead to many great discoveries. Theory of gravitation was formulated by Newton by his keen attention, fungal growth observed helped in the discovery of antibiotic penicillin by Alexander Fleming. Similarly signs and symptoms observed by Hippocrates laid the foundation of modern medicine. Attention leads to thinking, reasoning and further to learning. Poor attention leads to poor learning. Present concept of attention is that it is more careful observation. Primary red colour in "inverted red triangle" of family planning symbol is only for drawing **attention** that health care including family welfare facilities are available.

Perception denotes "observe, recognise and discriminate" the vision. Sound, taste, smell and touch help us to sense the stimulus. Thus perception is a behaviour where man interprets and appreciates. Heart attack patient who craves for fresh air to breath comes out with the perception that he gets good oxygen outside. Here, motivation and need makes him to do so though there is no difference in the air existing inside and outside, but the fact is that he lacks oxygen due to heart attack (myocardial infarction).

Perception (By Selection)

By value orientation (importance given) man perceives either accurately or otherwise. When a Nursing Superintendent instructs

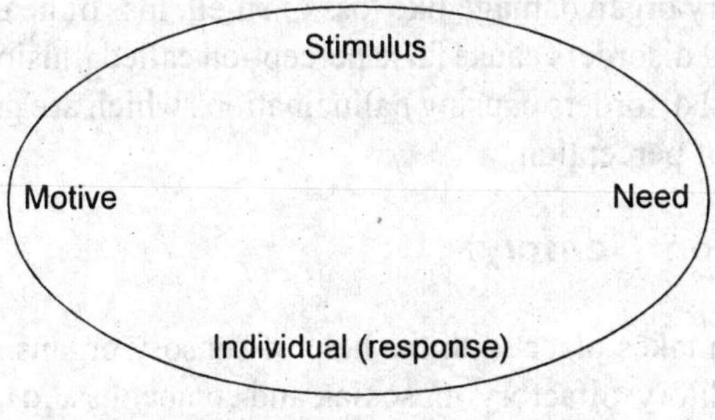

Figure 7.1: Perceptual organisation

a nurse, she does the job with immediate effect giving due importance. Suppose the same instruction is given by a neighbour or by an elderly person, accepting and perceiving are different. There is no value orientation that it must be done with immediate effect.

Perception (Emphasised)

There are many parts of perception; say early, middle and final parts. When man gives emphasis to final part, it becomes perception emphasised.

Perception (Introjected)

Many experiments have shown that memory of childhood has the ability of perception introjected. Neurosurgeon Penfield has shown that a scene "fire is engulfing parents" by a child is made available as perception but is taken off as this being not perceivable.

Determinants, duration and degree of attention and perception

Motivation, need and value system affect the duration and degree of attention and perception. Selectivity and emphasis enlarge the duration where as stability and introjections shorten the duration and degree of attention and perception. The determinants are:

a) Neurological causes
b) Psychological causes
c) Sensory organ damage like loss of smell, loss of hearing etc.
d) Mental disorders cause false perception called illusion
e) Mental disorders causing hallucinations which are gross error of perception.

Perception (Sensory)

Perception takes place with the help of sensory organs. They are visual, auditory, olfactory, muscular, and cutaneous and taste.

MOTIVATION

Motivation is the desire acquired to gratify the needs. It includes all activities and need which are directed to acquire gratification. Motivation is a driving force in human psychology. Man is driven to any social action by an inner force. Motivation thus is a best determinant of behaviour. There are two sides of motivation. They are:

1. Right doing behaviour called positive motivation.
2. Wrong doing behaviour called negative motivation.

Occasionally manipulation is confused with motivation. Manipulation is acquiring phenomenon for a developed desire and urge.

Biological motive

In health science we expect people to be self reliant on health related matters. This is expected of them to achieve improvement of health by their own effort called community participation. There are many issues related to biological motives like:

- Mother to attend antenatal clinic
- Child to be brought for immunisation
- Eligible couple to practice contraception
- Use of potable water to prevent water borne diseases.

Motivation Stages

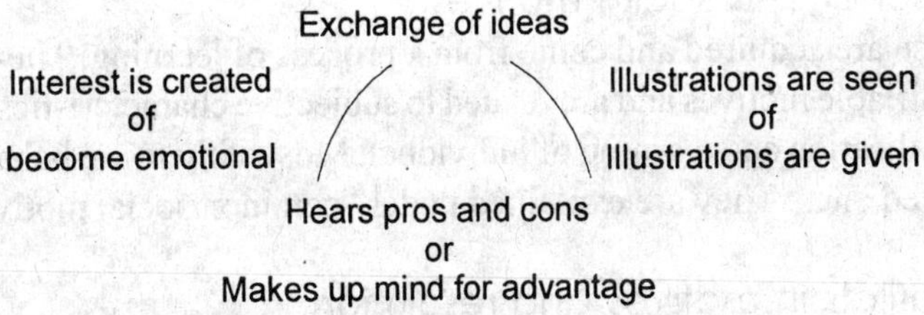

Figure 7.2: Stages of motivation

Typical example of stages of motivation is seen with another who has delivered recently in a hospital. Her peers exchange the idea of post partum tubectomy, which is easiest and comfortable. She sees other mothers getting satisfied with PPC programme and she sees more advantages if she avoids future pregnancy. She becomes emotional and gets motivated to undergo tubectomy at PPC ward.

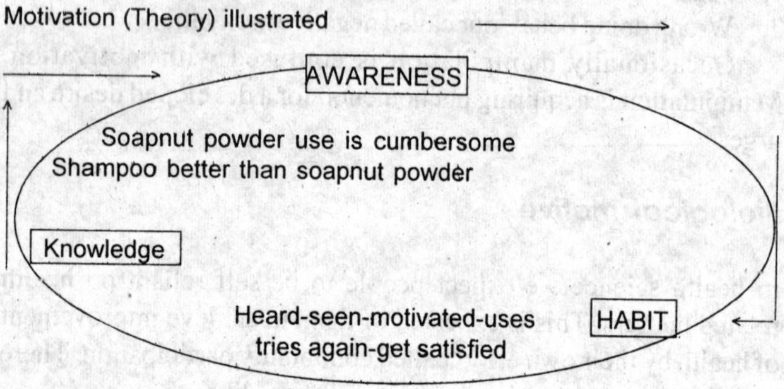

Figure 7.3: Trial-satisfaction-habit cycle

Habit is formed out of trial and satisfaction, which is out of motivation. Intense behaviour of motivation is produced by the curiosity. Then, a stable motivation is produced through self-life experience.

Personal and social motives:

These are acquired and come from a process of learning. They are modifiable motives and are related to subjective characteristics like socialisation and learning of individual. Most of them are behavior related ones. They are explained under "common social motives".

Conflicts in motives and resolution:

Motivation is deterred by many factors in psychological atmosphere of an individual or a group. These factors may take off the motive, which is called resolution. During the process, conflicts noted are:

- No good personal relations
- No good approach or free discussion
- Shortfall in guidance, support and encouragement
- No reward
- Unexpected bad vital event.

NEEDS AND DRIVE

Human needs are basic, additional and health needs. Some psychologists include luxury as a type of need. To acquire and gratify above needs man has two major types of drives. One is innate and the other acquired.

Needs are classified as under:

Social needs:
They are mainly desired needs like love, affection, recognition, education etc., which pertains to social nature of man.

Economic needs:
To fulfill the want of economic security is topmost need of the day.

Ego needs:
Self-respect, power, position and status are present updated item under needs.

Biological needs:
They are mainly survival nee ls like water, food, shelter etc.

Psychological needs:
They relate to desires that are attachments of animal kingdom. Sympathy, concern, achievement and influence are under psychological needs.

Drives, which are called motive, are classified as under:

a) Innate drive – They are desires to gratify the biological needs.
   i) Primitive innate drives have come from ancestors and are reflex oriented. To charge a man who beats you is similar to animal instinct.

  ii) Reflex innate drive like hunger contraction motivates to acquire food. Pavlov sees typical example with dog experiment.
  iii) Universal innate drive like acquiring a house, to become a good singer, like to have a baby boy, like to have an auto driven vehicle and so on.

b) Acquired drive – They are learned during social acts during the process of socialisation by a child or by an adult. A boy who wants to show off is acquired by observing other, dresses up most fashionably to meet a girl. This is an acquired drive to meet a psychological need.

Certain common social motives are always seen in a community. A girl without lower limb and upper limb is seen with a related behaviour to depend on another normal girl. This does not allow any other alternative but to have an acquired drive of "common social motive".

EMOTIONS

They are strong feelings of human beings. Emotions always motivate men, which are often irreversible. Visible changes of emotion are happiness, depression, anger, morose, hilarious etc. Invisible changes of emotion are rise in pulse rate, rise in respiratory rate, rise in BP, pain and tension. Both visible and invisible emotions usually return to normal with rest and relaxation.

- Specific emotions are — anger, fear, hate, and love
- Non specific emotions are — grief, joy, jealous, lust, moodiness, pity, sorrow and sympathy.

Emotions are major barriers of communication. Only after PASS OFF period of emotion, patient can talk freely and there is change of effective nurse-patient interaction for nursing procedures.

Thus emotion can be defined as *sudden force surfacing in the mind in response to a situation.*

Emotional states are positive and negative. Common illustrations are:

- Positive state of emotion — pleased, joyous, loved, satiated
- Negative state of emotion — sad, sorrow, anger, hatred, fearful.

Emotion as a motive:

Emotion expressed becomes a motive to gratify the needs. A nurse falling unconscious at work attracts attention. Her friends get emotional to see her condition. It is a motive for quick interaction. Duty nurse is motivated to attend to her at her best out of emotional attachment to her professional colleague. Both positive and negative emotions are found useful as motives in health care services.

Example of positive emotions as a motive:

– Very low birth interval with low birth weight show repeated infection. Emotionally it makes a mother to get motivated to accept spacing as contraceptive method for the sake of health of a newborn.

Example of negative emotion as a motive:

– Showing a clinical case of tetanus to a mother who used to resist TT for school children, explaining her that TT as the only weapon to prevent tetanus. Emotions of fear and concern in the mother allow her child to get TT by negative motivation.

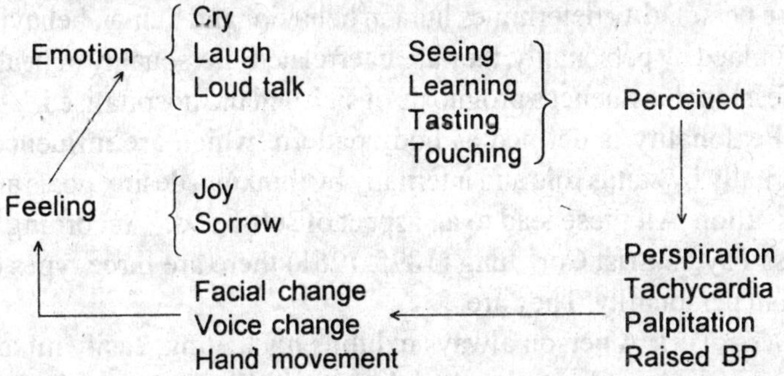

Figure 7.4: General theory of emotion

Emotion and culture are associated. Differences of emotions are seen in different societies, because the culture determines the way of expression of emotions.

Emotion and health

Various disorders are seen associated with emotions. These vary with age, sex and other demographic variables.

Adults	*Women*	*Children*
Loss of concentration	Anorexia nervosa	Tantrums
Loss of appetite	Amenorrhoea	Abdominal pain
Increased accidents	Pseudopregnancy	Spasms
Loss of sleep		Ticks
Palpitation		Aggressiveness

Control of emotions:

- By love, affection and appreciation among children
- By happy family life, reassurance, cultivating good habits, habit of reading, recreation
- Adaptation of philosophy of life, understanding one's own limitations and development
- Developing a sense of humour among adults.

PERSONALITY

Since personality determines human behavior and human behavior is moulded by personality, they are interrelated. Personality of health professional influences prognosis of sick and the hospitalised.

Personality is defined as body pattern, which are influenced externally by status role and internally by thinking, desire, goals and motivation. All these lead to an aspect of self-hood. According to Swiss Psychiatrist Corl Jung (1875-1961) there are three types of human personality. They are:

a) *Extrovert:* A person always exhibits his feeling, easily mixes, active, deemed practical and dare devil in action.

b) *Introvert:* A person always shy, keeps himself aloof and reserved.

c) *Mixed:* A combination of extrovert and introvert.

Personality development:

The factors help in development of personality are:

- Heredity (parents' reflection)

- Physical environment
- Social environment
- Gratified basic needs
- Attained educational level.

In human cycle, stage of a given cycle influence the development of personality:

Primary socialisation: infant and childhood
Secondary socialisation: school age child
Adventure, romance and love: adolescent
Mature and balanced: adult
Changes due to senescence: old age

Components of personality are tabulated as under.

Components	*Items*
Physical	Height, weight, skin colour, face
Emotional	Anger, fear, guilt, jealousy, love, worries
Intelligence	High I.Q.
Behaviour	Kind, affectionate, aggressive, submissive, balanced

Personality trait:

It is a stable personality manner and the tendency to behave in such a manner for a given social interaction. By 5 years and 10 months the child develops basic personality trait. In adulthood some traits are cultivated and some are concealed. Some of the examples of personality traits are:

- Kindness
- Reliability
- Sense of humour
- Loyalty
- Tactfulness
- Willingness to help
- Good manners
- Cheerfulness

Organisation of personality:

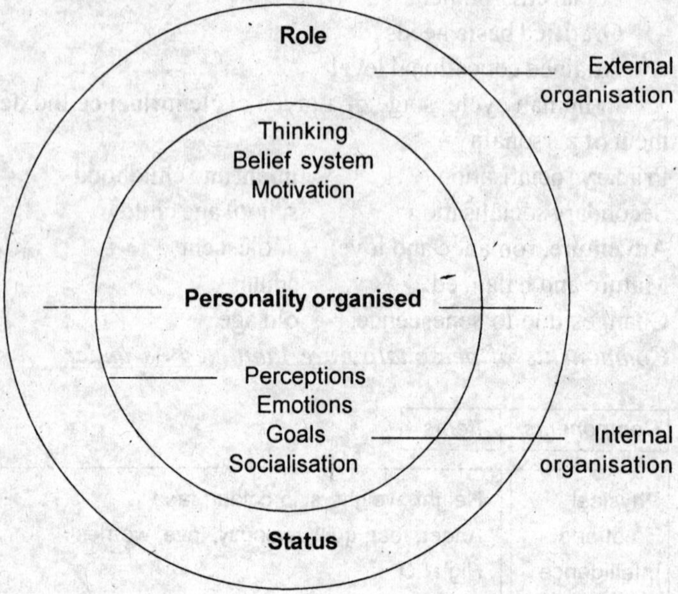

Figure 7.5: Organisation of personality

Theories of Personality

i. Theory of self: This is a basic feature of personality. Learning in the family setting and use of language contribute to development of personality. Socialisation within the family and foundation of attitude outside the family determine SELF. Self is symbolised with surname, family title, etc. Membership and class position extends the development of self.

ii. Kardiner's basic personality structure theory (Figure 7.6).

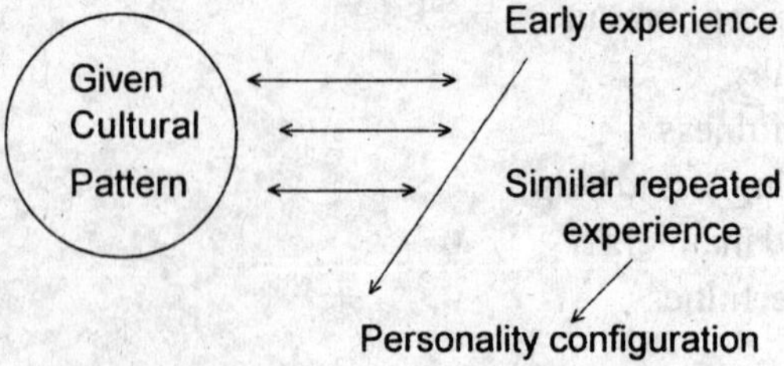

Figure 7.6: Kardiner's theory of basic personality

iii) Man's early life has a common and fundamental experience, which is reflected as "personality structure" and is a common phenomenon in any given society.
iv) Individuals will have many common elements in their personality that are common.
v) Early experience in life (of individual) varies from society to society. Hence personality norms also very from society to society.

Role of character in personality:

Character implies moral worth of an individual. It is different from personality. Character of an individual is variable from time to time whereas personality does not. Often conduct and character are synchronised. How a person conducts himself in a society is described in terms of character, though they mean differently.

Role of will in personality:

Determination of an individual forms a will. Willingness leads to a way in characterisation. Thus will and character are interdependent on each other. Will is transient and flexible which do not mould personality.

LEARNING

It is a psychosocial process that is required for survival and human progress. It is not equivalent to education but imply on acquiring knowledge, skills, and habit formation and perception development. Human intelligence has lead to a lot of changes in learning. Age-old observation and service at *Gurukula* for a learning, which used to take years of exposure has been reduced to a shorter spell of time where learning is processed even independently. Conscious learning is an adopted behavior where as unconscious learning is a conditional behavior.

Learning is an active and continuous process, which results in relatively permanent behavioral change in man. This is reflected through thinking, feeling, doing and attitude of a learner. It is also an outcome of one's interactive experience with his surrounding.

Law of learning:

It has come up through all stages of human development like birth, marriage, family formation, service, health, sickness, disability and even death. Learning is appropriated with survival and progress. It is for habit formation and perception development. Law of learning attains an individual to face any psychosocial interaction by reflex and do not allow him to succumb to injury or death.

Nature of learning:

Good deal of animal experiment and human experiment conducted by psychologists has brought out following aspects of learning:

- Reflex learning
- Learning by trial and error
- Learning by observation
- Learning by invitation
- Learning by doing
- Learning by remembering
- Learning by mental exploration
- Learning by any combination.

Principles of learning:

Various theories of learning have evolved certain principles, which are applied in learning activities to enhance learning. These principles are:

a) Human learning is guided by many set goals to achieve either at a shortest time or on a long term
b) Human needs in terms of physiological, safety, social esteem, self acculturation and aesthetic needs are strong reasons for learning
c) Life oriented education through observation and participation form the basis of learning

d) It is a voluntary process involving thinking, feeling and doing. Hence it involves the learner actively
e) Basic styles of leaning in man have been surface learning, deep learning and strategic learning
f) There should be learning with understanding which is called meaning orientation in learning
g) Learning leads to knowledge and in term should lead to application of mind
h) Learning should be for a real life situation and real life problem salvation
i) Learning should begin from known and should proceed to unknown
j) Reinforcement of learning is possible by feedback process.

Types of learning:

Present concept of classification of learning is described under taxonomy in education under a) cognitive domain, b) affective domain and c) psychomotor domain.

a. *Bloom's cognitive domain* (Figure 7.7):

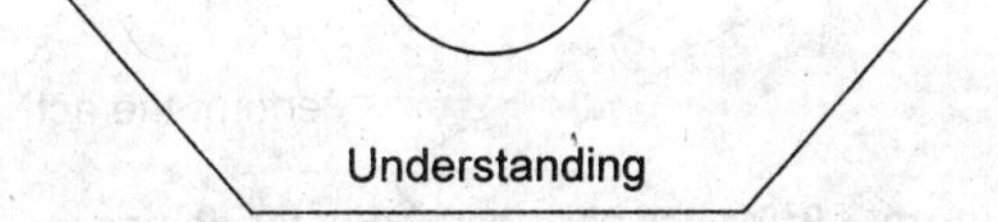

Figure 7.7: Bloom's cognitive domain of learning

b. *Bloom and Krathwohl's affective domain:*

This is the area of learning communication skills. It deals with interpersonal relationships. Learning is considered by interest, attitude, values, appreciations and adjustment. This is represented as a diagram in Figure 7.8.

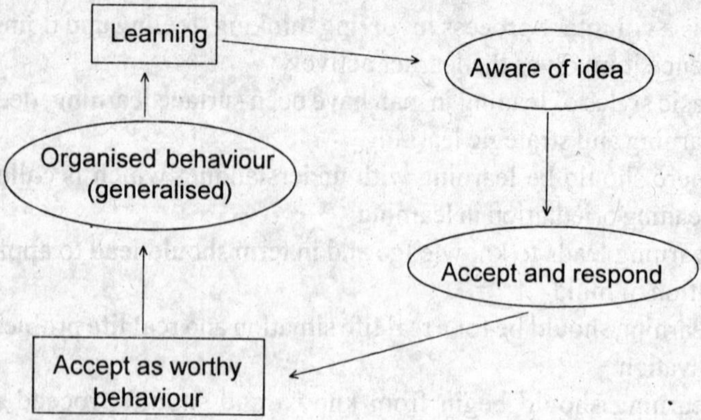

Figure 7.8: Affective domain of Bloom and Krathwohl

c. *Krathwohl's psychomotor domain:*

This is the area of practical skill learning. It involves mind and perception. Further human neuromuscular coordination determines this behavior of learning. It is represented as under:

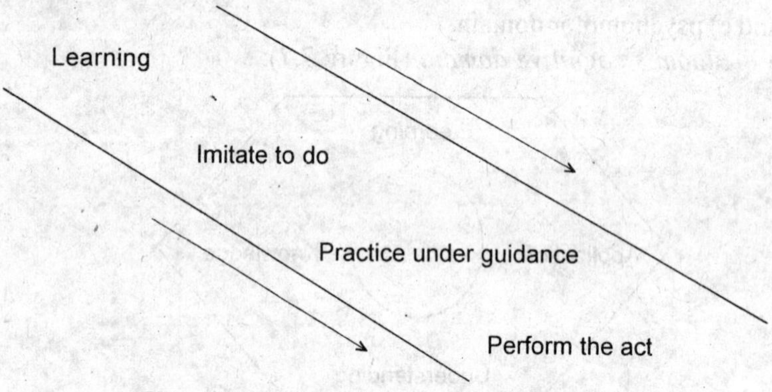

Figure 7.9: Krathwohl's psychomotor domain

Table 7.1: Examples for domains

Cognitive domain	Affective domain	Psychomotor domain
Nurse defines hypertension	Nurse understands anxiety of person going to OT for operation	Nurse learns and does Cardio pulmonary resuscitation

cont..

cont..

She enumerates Apgar score	She gives assurance to patient on the issue of scheduled operation	Nurse learns and gives enema to a patient as pre-operative procedure
She understands normal menses to decide ideal contraceptives	She helps to overcome emotion of patient to cooperate	

Effective learning is influenced by following factors:

Physical health	sick, deaf, blind, dumb
Mental health	worry, anxiety
Learning situation	facility, distance, material
Motivation	success, reward and gain
Intelligence	I Q level
Age	very young, very old

Theory of learning

Learning is a character, which differentiates human with other creatures. Man has great ability of learning. Various theories are postulated which are as under:

a) *Conditioning theory:*
According to Pavlov theory of conditioning response, learning involves a series of conditional responses. This is not relevant to the main learning process of sociology of nursing.

b) *Connectionism theory:*
According to Thorndike theory of connectionism is based on strengthening of bonds between stimuli and response (Fig: 7.10).

c) *Field theory:*
According to Gestalt, theory of Field considers the realisation of truth for the given situation. Learning in context is superior to learning in isolated parts.

d) *Learning model theory:*
According to Asubel, theory of learning model uses steps of problem solving for learning. It is better suited to nursing profession where clinical problem solving is used in case presentation and discussion.

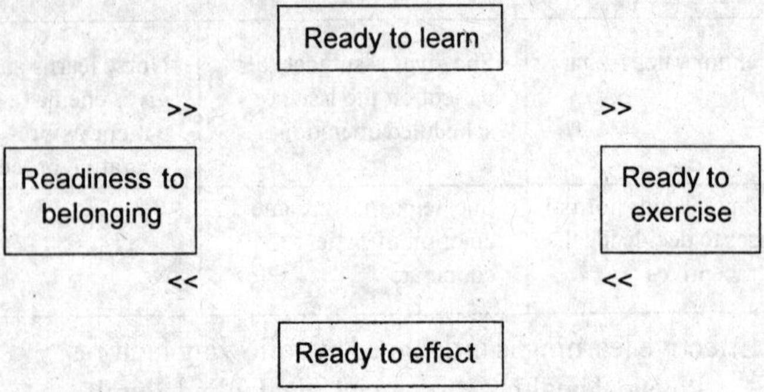

Figure 7.10: Connectionism theory of learning

Remembering and forgetting:

Thomas Addison has aptly said that:

"what we want to remember we easily forget and what we want to forget we easily remember" in his essay 'Art of forgetfulness'. Personality determines the way of remembrance and forgetting. Priority, closeness and benefit make the person to remember effectively. Remote items, general and nonbeneficiary make the person to forget easily.

Following Remembrance types are noted in human life:

- Innate or reflex based
- Routine based
- Inter related social based
- Vital event based
- Response based.

Regarding nature of remembering and forgetting, primary, secondary and re socialisation as well as psychosocial conflicts produce figures, words, and expressions of either remembering or forgetting. These psychosocial words are always purposive in nature. They try to serve a purpose of life situation. When man wants solace he remembers and forgets an event of considerable importance. Each minute, man gets flash of ideas, which cannot be equated to remembrance.

Religious discourse from Ramayana, Geetha, Quran, Bible is time immemorial slabs of remembrances learnt by-heart with a purpose. This remembrances and recitation itself can help an individual to forget unwanted memories of painful events. Thus remembering and forgetting are complimentary to each other.

THINKING AND REASONING

In man's perception, memory and imaginations have given way to thinking. As a higher order of mental process there is a psychosocial analysis in brain called reasoning.

Routine skill use, performance of an activity creates an opportunity for thinking.

Thinking may produce pleasant or violent aspect of thought. Outwardly expression of thinking is called extrovert and expressionless thinking is called introvert.

Bizarre thinking produces psychopaths in society.

Types of thinking:

a) *Objective thinking*
Here there is logical association between events and symbols. It is disciplined imagination. Objective thinking leads to many scientific innovations and discoveries.

b) *Wishful thinking*
Evading tendency of man leads to wishful thinking. It is also called Fantasies. This represents future anticipation of an individual. Very common wishful thinking are health and wealth. Among adolescents it is romance that make wishful thinking.

c) *Imaginative thinking*
Day dreaming and thinking of impossibilities like magic world or wonder world is imaginative thinking. This does not serve any purpose in life except spending time in an unfruitful way.

d) *Creative thinking*
It refers to thoughts brought out by an effective learning where there is scope for new ideas, new discoveries or new inventions. Creative thinking is a word used in dress making, art and painting.

Development of thinking

Education and commitment leads to development of objective thinking and creative thinking. Psychosocial norms should facilitate the process of required thinking and avoid unrequired thinking. Unrequired thinking leads to worrying which is not a healthy process. Hence required thinking should be allowed in an atmosphere of good psychosocial environment.

Camp lives, attending religious discourse; well-developed habits regulate a covert activity of objective thinking. Best thinking is to forget everything makes you and allow you to effectively regulate ways of your thinking.

Reasoning

It is the highest stage of human thinking where he tries to solve problems in life, which may be simple or complicated. Thinking and allowing the use of intelligence brings about reasoning. Careful reasoning disallows fallacies.

Types of reasoning

a) Primitive reasoning comes from conventional outline. Problem solving in daily routine are from primitive reasoning where individual's experience, family experience and society experience play a vital role.
b) Psychosocial reasoning comes from understanding of behavior, personality and interpersonal relationships.
c) Scientific reasoning is based on demonstrable scientific reasons in a reasoning.

PROBLEM SOLVING METHODS

Thinking and reasoning are used in solving both simple and complicated issues in life situations. Collection and arrangement of information on a subject, drawing conclusions and testing conclusions are methods used in practical problem solving methods.

Examples of problem solving by reasoning and thinking:

i) You are on a call to conduct normal home delivery in a house situated nearer the sub centre. When you visit the house, woman is in first stage of labour and there is rupture of amniotic fluid. Discuss your nursing line of management.

ii) An elderly woman at home has fallen and has sustained fracture of neck of femur (right side). Reason out your first line of management of this elderly woman at home.

iii) In labour room, you have conducted a normal delivery and the woman with newborn is to be shifted to postnatal ward. You are expected to assess the mother before shifting. Describe your nursing procedure (here the nurse is expected to explain post partum techniques to be performed viz., assessing the mother by:
- Palpating abdomen for fundus and bladder
- Evaluate the lochia
- Inspect the perineum
- Inspect and palpate the breast to confirm normalcy before shifting etc.

INTELLIGENCE

Intelligence is an aspect of personality. The act of intelligence include the process of:

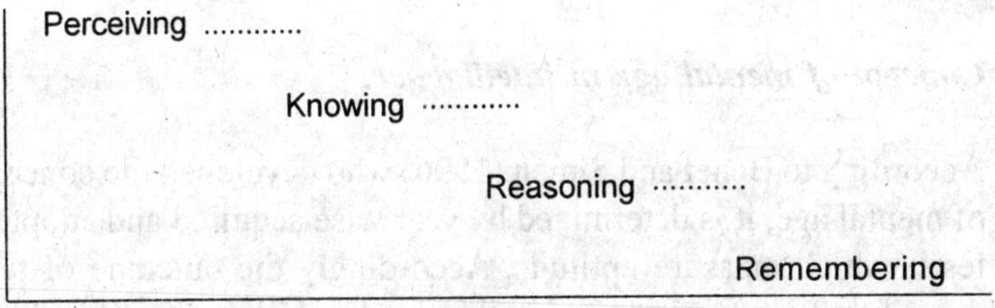

Figure 7.11: The process in intelligence

Intelligence is defined as " an ability to see meaningful relationships between interrelated matter".

Patient's subjective manifestations, patient's objective manifestations are to be observed, interpreted and nursing profession draws a meaningful decision.

General intelligence in nursing:

- Taking over charge
- Handing over charge
- Morning assessment before clinical round
- Attending to duty doctor's instruction and drug administration
- Sample dispatch for investigations
- Getting report collected
- Recording 4th hourly pulse
- 6th hourly respiratory rate
- 12th hourly body temperature
- 24th hourly B P

etc., are commonly done routine nursing which is managed with general intelligence.

Special intelligence in nursing:

- Assisting in heart transplant operation
- Performing kidney dialysis
- Case management in ICU, ICCU, IPCU

and emergency nursing care require special intelligence.

Concept of mental age in intelligence:

According to Benet and Simen (1896) who developed the concept of mental age, it is determined by year wise acquired and adopted tests, which measure aptitude. Accordingly the outcome of test describes the mental age or intelligence by skill. It did not include details of the lowered or altered mental acumen to group the child under normal for age or not normal for the age. A 7-year-old child passing intelligent skill test of child aged 6 year does not mean that the child is dull. This mental age determination serves as relative expression in psychoanalysis.

Concept of problem solving in intelligent test:

According to Terman who used abstract ideas for solving problems indicated that mental age is possibly determined. But it did not elicit adoptive behavior and motor ability properly.

Concept of intellectual development consideration for mental age:

According to Gessel who included four criteria to assess mental age described

- Motor ability
- Language development
- Adoptive behavior
- Personal social behavior

Gessel agrees that his concept has to be standardised.

Intelligence tests:

Devised by Binet and Simon and revised by Terman.

Individual performance test:

Understanding of language, general understanding, reasoning are used to measure psychological process of individual performance. Here time fixation is not a factor. There are specifications in test set to formulate evaluation of:

Young children
Illiterates
Feeble mindedness
Monolinguist.

I.Q. Tests applied which is a concept of mental age is improved upon to obtain a quotient by chronological age:

$$IQ = \frac{\text{Mental age}}{\text{Chronological age}} \times 100$$

Normal I Q range from 90 to 100 in our set up. When mental age and chronological age is same it comes to 100 which is an average.

e.g., $\frac{\text{Mental age}}{\text{Chronological age}} = \frac{9 \text{ years}}{9 \text{ years}} \times 100 = 100$

According to level of I Q grouping of individual is done which is as follows:

Level of intelligence	I Q
Genius	140 and above
Very superior	120 to 139
Superior	110 to 119
Normal	90 to 109
Low normal	80 to 89
Border line	70 to 79
Moron	50 to 69
Imbecile	25 to 49
Idiot	0 to 24

I Q measures the quality and potential intelligence. Higher performance is closely related to higher IQ.

Adult intelligence is analysied based on item analysis. According to Thurstone, adult intelligence includes 8 components and item analyses of these 8 components prove efficient method of intelligence analysis. They are:

- Memory of words and ideas
- Ability of finding out principles
- Ability of using principles in solving problems
- Ability of expression with appropriate words
- Ability of verbal comprehension
- Familiarity of elementary arithmetic
- Ability to perceive objects
- Flexibility and quickness of thought.

***Group performance tests*:**
Just as in examination, group test is administered to a group giving a specified time to complete. Here questions administered, tests the ability of group for perceiving, knowing, reasoning and remembering. Scoring system is adopted for ranking for best performance.

Uses of IQ in Psychology:
- Arrangement of special education to low IQ individuals
- Selection of able individuals for a given task performance
- To test the eligibility of individual for an entry to a formal or informal educations
- Help in work allotment according to ability of individual
- Common entrance tests for the selection to professional colleges
- Help in educational guidance
- Help in therapeutic prognosis.

Wing's comprehensive skill test:
It is a standardised measure of behavior, psychological function and social performance. This is known as HBS test (Wing's comprehensive Handicaps, Behavior and Skills Schedule). It details the scale for special abilities and disabilities. It is used as a research tool in psychoanalysis. A further extension of HBS is DAS where (Disability Assessment Schedule) mobility, communication and social interaction are measured in service contests.

EDUCATIONAL PSYCHOLOGY

From the early historic times, imparting knowledge from one generation to the next has been in vogue. In recent times the implication and relevance of education has undergone a revolutionary change due to the scientific and technological progress.

Proper education of child starts from birth and the child will be ready for formal education by 5 completed years of age. At this stage the child is still ready for learning only elementary things.

MEANING

Imparting sound education at different age level is an arduous task because intelligence development and level of ability is found to vary from age to age. Even children of same age are not alike in their mental capacity. The scientific study on individual differences has revealed that there is significant difference in the rate of mental growth and that different functions in the same child will grow at different rates.

Vijay aged 9 years is found able to solve arithmetic problems where as his elder sister Asha aged 12 years cannot solve arithmetic problem though she is more intelligent than Vijay. These variations in capacity render the problem of teaching even more difficult than it would otherwise be.

Personality and character is produced by education. Education gives place for more complex social adjustments and social responsibilities. Psychologists feel that education is for socioeconomic survival.

Scope and aim

In order to fit into a society man learned certain ways of life, as needed by a particular society. Thus objectives of education are determined by conditions outside the field of Psychology.

In the field of education, psychologist does not determine what is to be done. He points out the methods to be used in order to attain the desired result with the greatest degree of efficiency. In educational psychology main emphasis have been laid on child psychology, learning, special methods and personality. Of late, need for study of mental hygiene in educational psychology has been recognised and introduced in the study.

According to Kelly purposes of educational psychology are as under:

1. to give knowledge of the nature of the child
2. to give an understanding of the nature, aims and purpose of education
3. to give an understanding of the scientific methods and procedures which have been used in arriving at the facts and principles of educational psychology

4. to present the principles and techniques of learning and teaching
5. to give training in methods of measuring abilities and achievements in school subjects
6. to give knowledge on the growth and development of children
7. to assist in the better adjustment of children and help to prevent their maladjustment
8. to study the educational significance and the control of emotions
9. to give an understanding of the principles and techniques of character training.

Relation with other sphere

Children are admitted to the formal schooling at or after the age of 5 years. There may not be any psychological reason behind this. It is to secure more homogenous groups who can show similar grades by intelligent tests.

However, many dropouts are noticed from the school. Apart from psychological problems, there are non-psychological causes of dropouts. Philosophy, religion, politics, economic factors determine the scope of education. These areas may determine educational aims.

School curricula, which is older than psychology decides and determines the aims and objectives of education.

Extra curricular activities are necessary for all round education. This will help in getting social adjustment for the child.

Procedures and methods influence education. They are based on principles of psychology.

Individuals choose different careers, which will vary according to the interests, abilities and vocational plans of the students.

TEACHING METHODS

According to Monroe and Marks there are nine general teaching methods and are applicable to a wide variety of subjects. They are:

1.	The lecture method	Didactics and active lecturing
2.	The recitation method	Question by teacher, answer by pupil based on text book
3.	Object teaching	Observation of objects followed by comments by teacher
4.	Development method	Skillful question to help students to think through and clear up ideas
5.	The Laboratory method	Work with guidance in laboratory
6.	The Project method	Minimum teacher guidance only, group activity (student selection)
7.	The problem method	Problem assigned by teacher
8.	Socialised recitation	Democratic atmosphere by discussion in groups
9.	Teach and test until mastery (Unit mastery plan)	

Individual differences:

It is obvious that people are physically different. Motor and sensory functions also differ greatly in individuals. Based on individual difference in intelligence men are classified into genius, normal, idiot etc.

But scientific observation has made it clear that all are qualitatively alike mentally but differ in the degree of efficiency with which different functions work. Mind of a genius is similar to that of an idiot. But genius learns more easily, remembers easily and solves difficult problems.

Individual differences may divided within a group, into group differences including age sex etc., In one of the studies I Q of 100 nurses were analysed and following are the observations:

Mean I Q of 100 nurses = 102
S D of I Q of 100 nurses = 4.3

They are found distributed in the following manner:

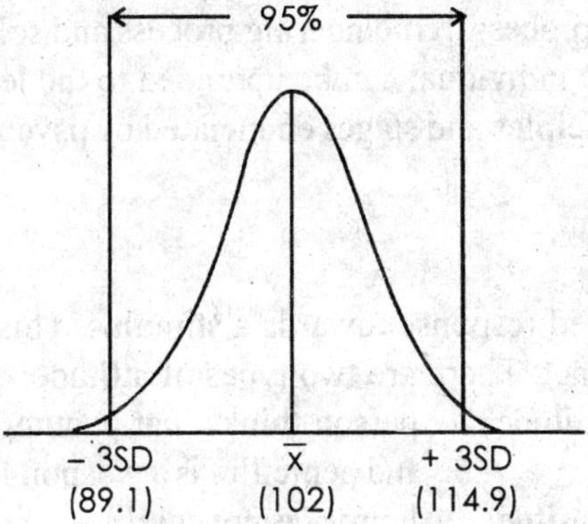

Figure 7.12: Normal distribution of IQ of 100 nurses

Since 99% of nurses in a normal distribution fall within 3 SD, 99% of nurses will have IQ between 89.1 to 114.9.

mean + or-35D = mean + 3 (4.3) = mean + 12.9

this comes to 102 plus or minus 12.9

therefore, 102-12.9 = 89.1

102 + 12.9 = 114.9

To get practical range of mental capacity of nurses, their age can be multiplied by 0.89 to get lower limit of distribution and by 1.15 to get upper limit of distribution.

Above finding points out that 99 out of 100 nurses will be having a range of IQ between 89.0 and 115. Modified and intensive teaching and training can improve those who are below 90.

HEREDITY AND ENVIRONMENT

They can influence individual difference like colour vision, state of memory, learning, deducing and reasoning. Group differences like age, sex etc., are usually influenced by environmental factors.

All individuals possess same grades of ability in learning, comprehension, performance etc. This leads us to deduce that all minds are qualitatively alike. But they are different in degrees of efficiency with which different functions work.

Learning process, remembering process and solving the problem by low IQ individual can be upgraded to the level of high IQ person by principles and stages enunciated by psychologists.

ATTITUDE

It is an expected response towards a stimulus. This describes the rudeness to react. There are two types of attitude:

1. Positive attitude — person thinks that pneumonia is curable and penicillin is a weapon for it
2. Negative attitude — leprosy is not curable

Attitudes signify individual preferences. They are acquired by social interactions and observed experiences. Attitude survey and attitude measurements are included in all present understanding of sociological phenomenon.

Development of attitude

Attitude is developed by experience and it is the effect of environmental stimuli. Attitudes are conditioned by the growth of intelligence. Examples of this are:

- Young child has limited capacity for understanding world and so are not capable of forming attitude
- 7-year child can observe a picture and make out what is happening in the picture. But it cannot interpret the reason for happening in the picture
- 12-year-old child can interpret the reason for what is happening in a picture
- Adolescence is marked especially by the secondary sexual characteristics and sex emotions.

Attitude development is influenced by:

- Home influences
- The social environment
- School environment
- Movie, TV serial

- Teacher
- The curriculum
- Teaching methods
- Group membership
- Associations

Measurement of attitude

Suitable scales are available to measure an attitude. A checklist prepared can be used to measure the attitude of a nurse, which is shown below:

Table 7.2: Attitude magerment scale

S.No	Items	Liked	Not liked	Not answering
1.	Present Nursing College Fee			
2.	Theory classes by Tutors			
3.	Demonstration by Matron			
4.	Dress code of Nurse			
5.	Shift duty by Nurse			
6.	SUPW by Nurse student etc.			

Instruction: Place a mark for your reaction

Teacher

One of the most importance factors in the mental make up of a person is his teachers' personality and behavior. A teacher should show a sense of fairness and justice, tact, sense of humor, good teaching skill and disciplinary practice.

Habit

They are accustomed way of doing things. They are acquired through repetitive act and are automatically exerted. Habits are exerted only under similar circumstances. They can become customs in due course to influence human behavior. They are grouped under

+ Good habits
+ Bad habits
+ Healthy habits

Principles involved in habit formation are:
- It starts from early childhood
- Frequently repeated
- Occurs in due course of time
- Emotions create habits
- They are under human control.

Conflicts

It is a powerful repulsive action between two courses of actions. They are configurated with emotions. Correction always keeps us away from conflicts. Conflicts cause emotional disturbances and leads to neurological disorders.

Frustrations

When man is unable to meet his needs and desire, he ends up with frustrations. External causes are failure, defeat, unemployment etc., and internal causes are poor health, low IQ etc.

Frustration can lead to nervous breakdown. Initially frustration is expressed as anger, dejection, hostility, suicidal tendencies.

Frustration leads to drug abuse and alcoholism.

Defence mechanism

Problems, failures, difficulties make a man to employ certain defence mechanism, which help him to get away to achieve happiness and success. Mentally healthy person uses them to achieve success or happiness. These defence mechanisms are:

a) Justification of behavior (Rationalisation)
   e.g., declaring grapes as sour
b) Blaming others for fault (Projection)
   e.g., Teachers are blamed for examination failure

c) Enhancing self esteem by compensation
   e.g., Poor in study show up as a good sports person
d) Escapism
   e.g., Pretend ill at examination
e) Displacing the situation
   e.g., Office problem reflected at home
f) Follow childhood practice
   e.g., Crying.

SOCIAL PSYCHOLOGY

It is a branch of psychology and deals with behavior of individual in society. It studies attitude of individual towards culture and social values.

GROUP BEHAVIOR

Interaction and social behavior of individual in a group is called group behavior. Custom, law and social obligations regulate man's activities. Group is lead by a leader. It is responsible for solidarity of the group behavior which is called *group morale.*

Group activity, group discussion, group opinion and group reaction are common psychosocial events in a society.

Group behavior can lead to progressive reformation of society or can lead to civil unrest.

Social group is responsible for primary, secondary and re-socialisation of an individual. Others share social attitudes in the community.

Group behaviour is the human response to health and illness that encompasses group dynamics and individual responses.

GROUP DYNAMICS

Community interaction in health care services, responses of community for illness particularly for social diseases, and self-help by the group in the society for good health constitute group dynamics.

Industrialisation:

It is the transformation of agricultural society into industrial society. By technical skill, man produces goods which are used in mass production of material.

Industrialisation is both social revolution as well as economic revolution.

There are social problems which arise out of industrialisation, which are:

- Slums and shanty town develops
- Water gets polluted
- Air gets polluted
- Lack of facilities for waste disposal
- TB, STD, Filaria, Malaria increases
- Food standard decreases
- Mental illness increases
- Road accidents increase
- Alcohol, prostitution and crime increases.

8

Psychiatry for Nurses

INTRODUCTION

In the sociological aspect of nursing, a nurse has a duty of very many complicated issues under mental health conditions where management of mental disorders, working of good practice in nursing care, understanding of hospital and community where role status, morale and leadership work upon her.

Mental health is poorly understood with regard to normalcy or abnormalcy and prescribes the word mad or not mad. If a person is not found adjustable then he is termed mad, which is not the case. Degree of health varies and no one is hundred percent healthy. Varying degrees of adjustments, understanding and ability to cope with emotional problems make a person normal and abnormal.

Criteria of an abnormal behavior (according to William C Menninges):

- Always worrying
- Unable to concentrate
- Unhappy without justified cause
- Very often and very easily loose temperament
- Regular insomnia
- Depression which makes incapacitated to fight
- Routine life is not normal

- Unnecessarily getting frightened
- Total disparity with always right and always wrong
- Somatic incurable pains and aches.

Defence Mechanism of Human Body

Sigmund Freud identified "Ego Defence Mechanisms" which are automatic unconscious response that help a person reduce painful feelings associated with emotional problems. It helps in:

- Protects from anxiety
- Insult is protected by self esteem
- Done or occurred at unconscious stage, it is a natural protective phenomenon
- It acts by denying mistakes, denying true motives and denying actions or impressions.

Common defence mechanisms are:

Repression:	forgetting unacceptable idea (under fits patient urinates which he cannot recollect a month later)
Sublimation:	Diverting unacceptable feeling (unmarried is dedicated to career)
Reaction formation:	Unconscious dealing for unacceptable desire (afraid of surgery patient jokes at it)
Dissociation:	Unconscious removal of painful experience (parents charred to death in front of a child and child cannot recollect it)
Conversion:	Change feelings to emotions {man does not want to marry gets fits [it is common hysteria]}
Rationalisation:	Give excuses (unconsciously) [a girl always seen seminude, when asked says that she can never find anything else to wear]
Projection:	Shift the blame on others (poor dancer blames floor level as unfit for dance)
Regression:	Childish behavior (anxious husband become completely dependent on wife, refusing to do even smallest thing for himself

Problem of mental disorders:

General behavior is changed	Loss of appetite
	Refusal of food
	Hostile
	Angry
	Gives up a job
	Restless
	Irrelevant talk
	Incoherent talk
	Obsession
Perception change	Illusion
	Hallucination
Memory change	Amnesia
Altered consciousness	Disorientation
Emotional disturbance	Mood change, depression
Motor activity change	Stupor
	Pathological imitations (ecopraxis)
	Immobile positions (catalepsy)

Common Mental Disorders Classified

I. Schizophrenia (split personality)
   Schizophrenia (simple)
   a. with positive symptoms
   b. with negative symptoms
   Paranoid schizophrenia [delusion + jealousy]
   Hebephrenic schizophrenia [disorganised]
   Catatonic schizophrenia [stupor or rigid]
   Residual schizophrenia [eccentric]
   Undifferentiated schizophrenia
II. Maniac depressive psychosis [excitement or depression]
   Hypomania
   Manic excitement
III. Paranoia
   Psychoneurosis
   Character disorders

Therapeutic Nurse Patient Relationship

Therapeutic relation starts with giving possible attention for "nursing care of whole patient" which refers to body and mind, is key to success for overcoming physical and emotional difficulties. Patient's new social attachment to ward may not be overlooked.

There is a need to offer nursing care in private in order to spare sensitive patients the distress of watching and being observed.

Nursing staff creates the feeling of relation (optimism). Strain (pessimism) is also possible in her nursing role.

In recent years the atmosphere in children ward and geriatric ward are receiving much attention. The pathetic loneliness of the aged when they are in bed is a handicap to recovery. Deafness, shortsightedness and inhibited movements make it too difficult to bridge the conventional distance of beds. Playrooms for each child patient are an advantage in case of paediatric ward. In mental hospitals the therapeutic effect of group treatment where, use of patients' ability to help each other has been found immensely helpful.

The term "therapeutic community" was originally coined to describe how in a particular hospital for psychopathic patients, a community spirit developed which helped many patients to gain self respect, to cultivate their assets to the fullest degree and to gain control over their antisocial and aggressive tendencies.

Understanding of the stages of motivation helps the overture to such important matters as toilet training, weaning, feeding, play, education etc., among child patients.

Psychoanalytic Model

Therapeutic nursing involves many activities that will improve health care. Following are the basis of an effective therapeutic nursing care. They are:

- Always sickness is associated with psychological basis
- Treatment by drugs, injections, operations alone are not sufficient
- Sympathy, care, comfort are part of treatment of any illness

- Emotional problems should be understood and should be taken care of
- Nurse should understand that three factors influence any physical illness and they being
  - the patient
  - the illness
  - the social environment

  Hence there is a need for holistic approach.
- Psychotherapy is required to patients, paramedical and medical service givers
- Psychological comfort and care of relatives should be attended.

Behavioral Model

Conscious mind has all awareness. Subconscious mind comprises memories that can be brought out. Unconsciousness mind contains memories which cannot be recalled. So psychoanalysis of behavior is possible by:

a. Free association
b. Dream analysis

The interacting system according to Freud's theory are:

a. Id
b. Ego
c. Super ego

They are primitive, reality based and controlled mind respectively.

Psychosomatic Disorders

They are group of disorders in which emotional factors have a demonstrable role in the aetiology. All of them are stress related disorders.

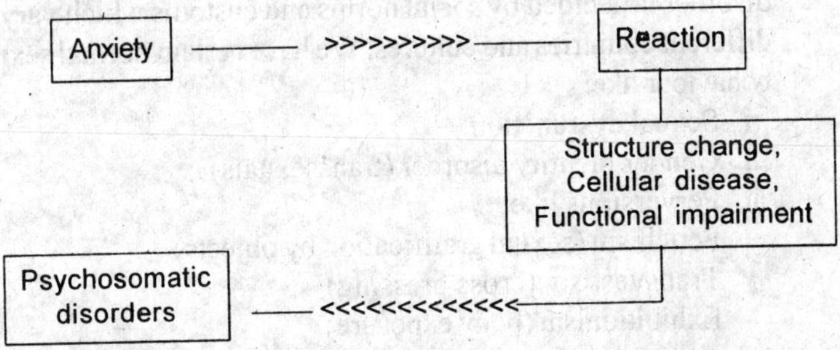

Figure 8.1: Progression path of psychosomatic disorders

Table 8.1: Common causes for psychosomatic disorders

Common psychosomatic disorders are	Common causes could be
High blood pressure	Response to emotion
Asthma	Personality traits
Peptic ulcer	Family pattern
Ulcerative colitis	Prolonged stress
Irritable bowel syndrome	
Arthritis	
Headache	
Eczema	
Diabetes	
Anorexia nervosa	
Obesity	
Psychogenic pain	

Management of these psychosomatic disorders are:

- Good therapeutic relationship
- Encourage the patient to discuss his problems
- Create a feeling of acceptance
- Encourage family participation in therapy
- Teach relaxation exercises.

An Individual in Our Society with Characteristic Disorders

a. *Sexual disorders:* It is difficult to define it because the disorder is decided by social norms and customs which vary in different countries and cultures. We have certain normal sexual behaviour like:

i. Sexual dysfunction
ii. Gender identity disorder (transsexuals)
iii. Perversions like
Fetichism (sexual gratification by objects)
Transvestism (cross dressing)
Exhibitionism (body exposure)
Voyeurism (peep undressing)

Paedophilia (child sex)
Sexual sadism (inflicting pain)
Sexual masochism (seek beaten)

b. *Alcohol and substance dependance:* Alcohol withdrawal delirium occurs in 5% of alcoholics who stop alcohol. Correction of dehydration, electrolyte imbalance, control of fits are to be attended along with careful monitoring of vital signs.

Opioids, antipsychotic drugs show involuntary muscle contractions ending with stiffneck, stiff mouth, elevated eyeball.

Care has to be exerted with psychiatric emergencies during special nursing care of in patients.

c. *Sociopath reaction:* Antisocial, cruel minded personality needs attention of safety, security and its management is similar to psychiatric emergency.

d. *Childhood disorders:* Proportion of childhood mental disorders can be gauged by the fact that they constitute 38 to 40% of our population which comes to about 390 million at present, as per 2001 census.

Common causes of disorders are biological causes like hereditary, illness; psychological causes like broken homes and social causes like poverty.

Common illness are: Mental retardation
Autism (driven to fantasy)
Conduct disorders
Specific developmental disorders
Personality development disorders
Hyperkinetic disorders
Tics
Mannerism

Basic responsibility of nurse should be based on the recognition of following features:

- Child behavior not appropriate to age
- Child behavior lead to disability
- It is against social expectations

Hence, apart from carrying out instructions for therapy, a nurse need to do the following:

- Obtain details of problem
- Explain parents
- Assurance to parents
- Play therapy.

Modern Therapy in psychiatry

Treatment of mentally ill health patient is not specific since it varies from person to person. Nurse being closer to patient, has important role in social therapy, psychological therapy and nursing therapy. Her action, attitude and skills to help patient to deal with his problems are themselves an essential part of his treatment. They can be tabulated as under:

Table 8.2: Modern therapy in psychiatry

Therapy	Examples
Physical therapy	Drug therapy, ECT, psychosurgery
Psycho pharma-cology	Psychotherapy of individual, group, family
Hypnosis	By altered state of consciousness induced by conditioning and skilled use of suggestions
Play therapy	Very helpful for young and the old. Diversion by play can get over tension and anxiety.
Activity therapy	Occupational, music, dance, psychodrama, recreation and psychosocial therapies

Crisis Situation

It is also called crisis intervention, which is a type of brief psychological method of treatment for the person who is in an emotional crisis. Crisis is a sudden event in one's life that disturbs the mental equilibrium during which the usual coping mechanisms fail.

Grief is a crisis, which normally does not require intervention. Reassurance, suggestion and environmental manipulation are found sufficient. In some cases it may require psychotropic medication.

Suicide is an emergency crisis, which needs one or two sessions of treatment. If necessary hospitalisation may be necessary. It is possible to prevent suicide by behavioral therapy and relaxation therapy.

Community Psychiatry

It is a branch of psychiatry that develops and maintains organised programs for the prevention, promotion and rehabilitation of mentally ill person.

In a defined population, care given through health workers and community health guide for a continuous care and integrated with regular health service is called community mental health care.

Table 8.3: Levels of community mental health care

Primary Prevention
– Elimination of causative agent – Reducing risk factors – Enhancing man's resistance – Reducing stress – Counselling like student counselling, marriage counselling, sex counselling genetic counselling etc. – Mental health education
Secondary Prevention
– Population screening – Crisis intervention service centres are established – Health awareness for early diagnosis
Tertiary Prevention
– Rehabilitation after defects noticed

The nurse in mental health nursing: It is now well established that it is not just diagnosis and treatment, but require promotion and reservation of good mental health. There are many areas where mental health nursing play vital role. They are:

- Early diagnosis, prompt treatment
- Rehabilitation
- Group psychotherapy
- Individual psychotherapy
- Mental health education
- Use of psychoactive drugs
- Follow up services.

9

Anthropology for Nurses

INTRODUCTION

Anthropology is one of the science that determines human behavior and hence is a specific branch of behavioral science. Anthropology is the scientific study of man through his physical, social and cultural aspect.

The goal of anthropology is to provide a holistic account of humans and human nature.

Biological anthropology includes the study of human evolution, human evolutionary biology, population genetics.

Cultural anthropology is often based on ethnography, a kind of writing used throughout anthropology to present data on a particular people. The study of kinship and social organization is a central focus of cultural anthropology

Archeology is the study of human material culture, including older pieces of human culture

Linguistics is the study of language which seeks to understand the process of human communication.

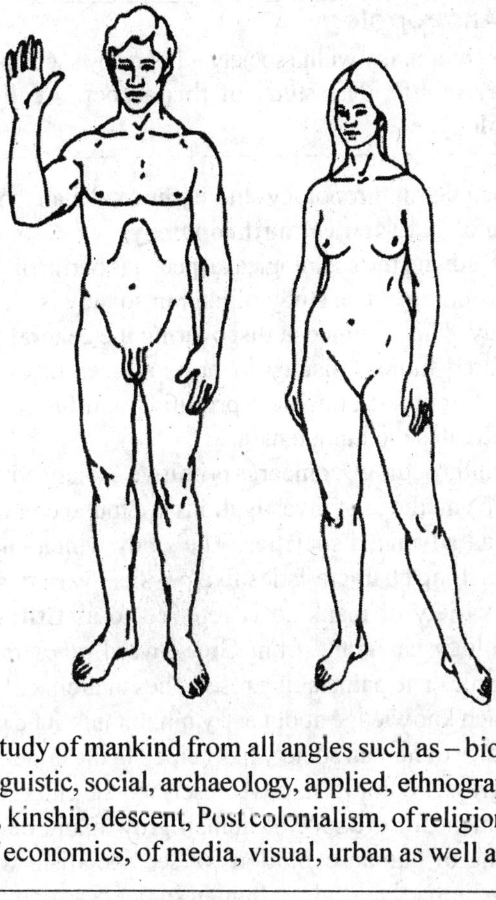

Scientific study of mankind from all angles such as – biological, cultural, linguistic, social, archaeology, applied, ethnography, archeology, kinship, descent, Post colonialism, of religion, of ecology, of economics, of media, visual, urban as well as medical.

Physical Anthropology

It deals with the human evolution, human racial differences and inherited human characteristics. The inherited character is through bodily traits are studied. Human cycle by his growth and course of his life span which are available by scientific observation is called **Physical Anthropology.**

Cultural Anthropology

Man has the capability to think, feel, act and behave and his ways of doing influence them. The study of these human activities is called **Cultural anthropology.**

Social Anthropology

Man in his community within society is bound by social boundaries, social way of life. The study of this aspect is called **Social anthropology.**

Thus, as a science anthropology studies the total man, both in health and disease called **Medical anthropology.**

While studying the sociological aspect it is pertinent to highlight social anthropology. The study of man in society is an expression for sociology. This is aimed at discovering the general laws which have regulated human history in previous centuries. When we compare different societies with primitive non literate society, it again investigates the human nature.

Social anthropology compares primitive society with advanced societies. The methods of investigations are found common to both primitive and advanced societies. The study which enquires into the distinguishing characteristics like physical variety of mankind and moral variety of mankind is referred to as **Ethnology.** The word Ethnology has come from Greek word *ethos* meaning the study of people. The painstaking researches of archaeologists have given us much knowledge about early inhabitants. The great diversity in the form of human society has helped in the understanding of human progress. Sociologists have described the emergence of law and government for the sake of human growth and development. In the tracing of human evolution we see socialism which deals with positive inductive study of human society.

In the beginning of this century the social anthropology was engaging the specific philosophical enquiry into human progress. Here Institutions, customs and beliefs were also taken note of. In early part of social anthropology the order of development of techniques are found not much advanced.

As a part of natural development and natural origin, progress of mankind saw language, law and religion. This gave an impetus to the act of reasoning in human beings. From 1870, the beginning of social anthropology must have been started. It gained impetus in exploring similarities of social features in different regions. Taylor

exploring similarities of social features in different regions. Taylor depicted the beliefs of man in life and its survival after death. McLennan described *totemism*, a custom associated activities. Speculations under social anthropology can mask the scientific study. For example, matriarchal speculation is found to mask the study of kinship in the family. In some of the sectors of Kerala (India) female line is following in inheritance of property and succession. A man related to his mother's brother found inheriting position and possession of his mother's brother. Here relationship of father and child is not recognised.

In social anthropology two concepts ***social structure*** and ***social organisation*** need mentioning. Structure refers to arrangement of persons and organisation refers to activities.

10

Applied Sociology

INTRODUCTION

Industrial revolution and scientific revolution of past 2 centuries, showed the advancement of sociology to the extent that it went out of our reach. It included every inch of present political system of the society. Theoretical debate is going on as to its placement for adopting principles and practices of natural sciences. Thus we have come across sociological positivists and anti positivists in this debate, both contributing to the application of sociology to the present Development of Science and Technology.

The science of sociology has brought a vivid picture to the world of social problems like alcoholism, drug abuse, prostitution and the like. It also provided the measures say social measures through social policy to check the menace from social problems.

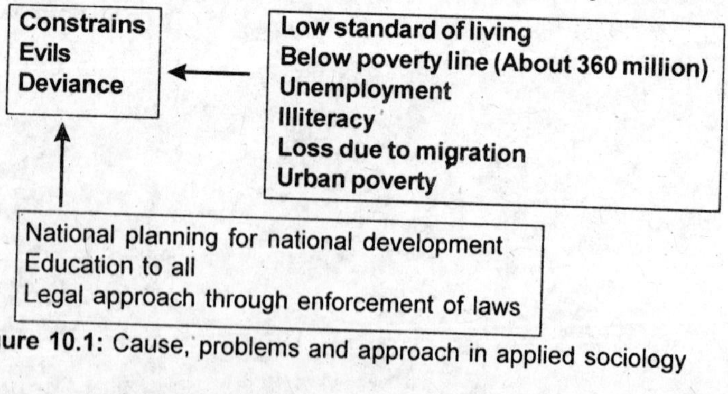

Figure 10.1: Cause, problems and approach in applied sociology

Of late many social organisations joined to provide social welfare activities apart from the governmental social welfare schemes and activities in the country. Thus the contribution of sociology is social assistance, social defence and social insurance through social security activities. These revolutions have changed the world trend both in developed countries and developing countries.

SOCIAL PROBLEMS

All of us follow social norms, which is the outcome of socialisation, which we are used to doing so. All social norms are accompanied by sanctions that promote conformity and protect against non-conformity. A sanction is any reaction from others to the behavior of an individual or a group that is meant to ensure compliance with a given norm. There are some individuals who refuse to live by the rules that majority of us follow. We come across alcoholism, drug users, sexually transmitted diseases, juvenile delinquency, prostitution and violent criminals. These people do not show confirmatory to a given set of norms that are accepted by significant number of people in a community. Some have health implications in the community.

Table 10.1: Common social problems in a society

Social evils	Social deviants	Other social problems
Alcoholism Caste system Gender discrimination Child abuse Corruption Prostitution	Drug abuse Juvenile Delinquency Suicide	Sexually transmitted Diseases Violent criminals Unmarried mothers Physically challenged

Social Evils:

1. Alcoholism

Alcoholism is a global health problem. Over the past 50 years production, consumption and abuse has grown to such an extent to cause civil unrest. With the changes in social order alcohol is being considered as a symbol of civilisation resulting in more alcohol abuse. Mild to serious health problems are observed due to alcoholism:

They are:

- loosing balance by poor reasoning due to alcohol content in the blood
- peptic ulcer
- gastritis
- cirrhosis of liver
- hypertension
- heart failure
- urinary disturbances
- impotence and sterility
- foetal damage.

Social implications of alcoholism are as under:

- crime
- murder
- prostitution
- family negligence
- unemployment
- indebtedness
- malnutrition
- delinquent child
- traffic accidents
- other psychosocial problems.

Health education and awareness programme can check the menace due to alcoholism. There are de-addiction centres to rehabilitate alcoholics. Simultaneously they need good and continuous counselling.

2. ***Caste System***
3. ***Gender Discrimination***
4. ***Child Abuse***
5. ***Corruption***
6. ***Prostitution***

It is one of the oldest known social evils very commonly seen in broken homes, illegitimate love making, easy money as sex worker and poverty etc., Poverty seems to lead a woman to prostitution.

Prostitution is closely related to sexually transmitted diseases and AIDS.

Social regulation and a good culture in the family can reduce its incidence. The suppression of Immoral Traffic Act in Women and Girls (SITA) 1956, now called as the Immoral Traffic (Prevention) Act 1986 covers men and women who are exploited for commercial purpose.

Remedy for social evils:

- Health education
- Socio economic development plans
- Rehabilitation with de addiction programmes.

Social Deviants

1. Drug Abuse

Drug users

Repeated intake of habit forming drugs cause drug addiction. Now it is called as substance abuse. Patient show violent behavior like nausea, vomiting and other severe allergic manifestations if a given drug is not made available. This is called physical dependence. Gradually drug users increase their dose intake indicating the development of tolerance. Finally they even commit crime by compulsion to procure drug.

Social factors, which seem to influence drug abuse are:

- accessibility to young generation
- broken home
- disturbed home environment
- escapism from tension life and frustrated life

Common drugs seem to produce drug abuse are:

Table 10.2: Drug abuse substances

Narcotics	Morphine Heroin Codeine opium
Marijuana	Hashish Ganja Bhang
Hallucinogens	L S D Mescaline
Hypnotics	Barbiturates
Tranquillisers	Chlorpromazine Equanil
Stimulants	Amphetamine Cocaine

Case management

Drug identification
De-toxication in hospital environment
Counselling
Rehabilitation
Change of environment in some cases
Psychotherapy in some cases

Social therapy

Individual health education
Target group awareness

Legislation:

Narcotic Drug and Psychotropic Substance Act 1985
Combating the source

2. *Juvenile Delinquency*

Delinquent mean any person who is deviated from his or her normal behavior, thus committing theft, sexual offence, murder or burglary.

Juvenile delinquency means problem with children. Broken homes, poverty, feeble minded children precipitate the child to commit an offence. Here juvenile crime is confined to a boy below 16 years and a girl below 18 years of age.

Social measures like improving family life, free schooling for education, child guidance and other social welfare services are aimed at preventing juvenile delinquency. The children Act, 1960, provide legislative measures through orphanage, foster home, adoption, borstals and remand homes. Of late, Juvenile Justice Act 1986, gives room for rehabilitation of Juvenile delinquent.

3. *Suicide:*

Low skills, low training, low education, poor personality development, loss of money, loss of material, loss of job may lead to suicidal tendencies.

Measures for social deviants:

- Health education
- Intervention
- Rehabilitation

Other Social Problems

1. *Sexually transmitted diseases (STD)*

The STD is associated with creation of slum and shantytown. Industrialization influence sexually transmitted diseases.

STD and prostitution are interrelated. In early days 5 classical venereal diseases viz., *syphilis, gonorrhoea, chancroid, Lymphogranuloma venereum* and *Granuloma Inguinale* used to top the list. Now, more than 20 different entities are included in the list of STD. Among new entrants genital chlamydial infection, genital herpes, genital human papilloma infection and AIDS are found to be predominating.

Social causes of STD are many and following are commonly seen in predisposing to infection:

a) prostitution
b) possible high financial return
c) conducive life-style of urbanisation
d) idea of independence leading to behavioral change
e) alcoholism
f) broken homes.

Case detection by screening, full course of treatment of diagnosed cases; health education of the community seems to be practicable intervention strategies.

2. *Violent criminals*

Various causes including lack of social regulations in the family and mental illness due to organic lesions found to produce violent criminals. Little different to crime, we have deviant. The concept of deviant is much broader than that of crime, which refers to nonconformist, conduct that break law.

3. *Unmarried mothers*

It is insignificant in developing countries like India. But teenage mothers out of wedlock issues are becoming social problems.

They require guidance, counselling and nursing care.

4. *Physically challenged*

Now, this category comprising of blind, deaf, physically handicapped, crippled with leprosy, mental retardation are included under social problems.

Rehabilitation services with health care education of blind, deaf, physical rehabilitation, vocational training are being undertaken to meet the above social challenges.

SOCIAL SECURITY

Social security is defined as "security that society furnishes through appropriate organizations, against risk to which people are exposed". Common risks are

- Sickness
- Invalidity
- Maternity
- Old age
- Death

Social security is classified under three categories:

a) for industry workers	Indian Factory Act, 1948 ESIS, 1948 Workman Compensation Act, 1923 Central Maternal Benefit Act, 1961 Maternity Bencfit Acts of State (1929 to 1948) Family Pension Scheme, 1971 Coal Miners' PF and Bonus Scheme Act, 1948.
b) for civil servants	Pension Gratuity (Payment of Gratuity Act 1972) Contributory Health Services Scheme, 1954 Provident Fund Employees' PF Act, 1952 Family Pension Central Government Health Scheme, 1963

c) for public

Insurance schemes
State Old Age Pension Acts
Old Age Pension Scheme, 1995
PPF.

Social security benefits are distributed through three channels. They are:

Table 10.3: Types of social security

Social assistance It includes old age pension, widow pension, assistance to leprosy patients, Family planning assistance, old age homes, and stipend for unemployed graduates, maternity assistance to the poor and facility for senior citizens.
Social defence It includes punishment of criminals, Anti Dowry Act, eradication of beggary, welfare of prisoners, alcohol prohibition, gambling control, prostitution control and suicide counselling.
Social insurance It includes ESI, crop insurance, accident insurance, insurance for health etc.

SOCIAL AGENCIES

As part of socio cultural tradition, there are many social welfare services as an integral part of community development. In the field of social welfare, it is estimated that there are about 60000 voluntary organisations in India doing yeomen services. Coordination of social welfare is by Ministry of Social Welfare and Central Social Welfare Board. They are categorised as:

1. General welfare activities
2. Women welfare activities
3. Child welfare activities
4. Specific disease control
5. Specific welfare activities.

Social welfare is now closely linked with social policy, both at government and state level organisations. Through social policies welfare is delivered to the public. India is becoming welfare state in the sense that it is ensuring a minimum standard of living for all people as a right of citizenship. It is trying to provide economic justice and equalities.

Factory Act in many occupational placements also introduces the welfare to its work force.

Welfare of the old people is taken up by social organisations. Some of the welfare activities for the aged being taken up in India are:

- Home care of aged sick
- Meals on wheels supply of low cost or free meals
- Hospital conveyance to the sick, similar to pregnant woman in rural areas
- Performance of household chores by home help
- Companionship to the lonely old.

SOCIAL HYGIENE

In an unrest society the causes are found to be social problems. They are to be tackled to overcome unrest. Health personnel including doctors and nurses opine that social arena is a fitting Dias to tackle the problem of unrest.

Thus social hygiene started assisting public health through policies for arranging minimum needs of the society. The policy directed for attending social hygiene through following components:

- Rural health
- Rural water supply
- Rural electrification
- Elementary education
- Adult education
- Nutrition
- Environmental improvement of urban slums

- Homes for landless labourers.

The objective of this was to provide basic minimum needs and thereby improve the living standards of the society. Actually social hygiene is the expression of the government for social development and economic development of people particularly the under privileged and underserved population.

Historically we come across the condemnation of low wage scales, which are fundamental cause of ill health. Mortality and disease are proportional to the degree of poverty, poor education and criminality.

First guarantee of health of a newborn is the health of its parents. Ancient people had this in their mind but they could not take steps to prevent marriages of people with hereditary disorders. Thus marriage guidance and marriage counselling have their role in preventive steps. Under Reproductive and Child Health programme we have:

- Reproductive health
- Maternal health
- Child health.

Similarly school children do need basic requirement like building, chair-desk, good light, ventilation, lavatories and sanitary installations. The ongoing school health service programmes have taken cognizance of these needs.

Social illnesses like Tuberculosis and leprosy needed much attention of social hygiene. Myths underlying diseases causation was to be tackled. All misconceptions had to be removed to see that these diseases also are similar to any other diseases in their occurrence through multifactorial causation.

With the exception of mental deficiency, diseases like psychological disturbances, neurosis, psychoneurosis and specific mental diseases can often be forestalled by current mental hygiene. Diagnosis and treatment combined with an effect of re-adoption make the cure possible.

Various clinics have helped in adaptation of social hygiene under above circumstances.

Alcohol and drug abuse need attention through social hygiene. Public attention drawing and creating awareness on the ill effects of alcoholism and drug abuse have been found useful in tackling these social problems.

Increased life expectancy and decreased birth rate have created problems of old age and created the need for pre old age specific programmes. Social hygiene, medicine and social policy will help in suitably tackling the above problems.

Social hygiene was hitherto passive, defensive and negative. But today it is active constructive and positive to show better life as well as means of harnessing nature to human ends.

SOCIAL WELFARE PROGRAMMES

1. Minimum Need Programme

Started in 1974 to provide basic needs of the society and to improve living standard of people.

It is the social and economic development of the country particularly the underprivileged and underserved population. This provides:

- Rural health
- Rural water supply
- Rural electrification
- Elementary education
- Adult education
- Nutrition
- Environment improvement of slums
- Houses for landless.

1 PHC for 30000 population (200000 tribal and hilly)
1 sub centre for 5000 population (3000 tribal and hilly)
1 Community Helath centre for 1 lakh or for 1 community development block.

2. 20-point programme

Started in 1975, restructured in 1986 with the objectives of:
- Poverty eradication
- Raising productivity
- Reducing inequalities
- Removing social disparity
- Improving quality of life.

Started in 2000 to overcome poverty and social disparity. Government of India has adopted the U.N. Millennium Development goals in seven areas. They are:

1) Provision of peace, security and disarmament
2) Development and poverty eradication
3) Protecting our common environment
4) Protecting human rights, democracy and good governance
5) Protecting the vulnerable
6) Meeting the special needs of developing countries
7) Strengthening the United Nations.

India has set the following health related Millennium Development Goals:

1) Eradicate extreme poverty and hunger
2) Reduce child mortality
3) Improve maternal health
4) Combat HIC/AIDS, malaria and other diseases
5) Improve environmental sustainability
6) Develop global partnership for development
7) Ensure environmental sustainability
8) Develop global partnership for development.

11

Social Responsibility

Health care is a team work. The team include professional and auxiliary health personnel who are needed to give health care. Nursing care is nearly 50% of health care in the context of care, control and social responsibilities.

Maintaining the Individuality of Man

A patient is an individual member of society who has rights, privileges and immunities which would be respected regardless of his race, creed, social or economic status and personal fears and needs which usually are exaggerated by his illness.

Expected functions of professional care are:

- Care of the sick
- Care of the injured
- Prevention of diseases
- Promotion of health
- Diagnosis
- Treatment
- Rehabilitation
- Vocational training
- Health education and health awareness
- Research for appropriate technology.

Social responsibilities are laid down by the Ministry of Health and FW services in the job responsibilities of health workers in the health system of the country.

Social responsibilities of health assistant female are:

1. Supervision and guidance
2. Teamwork
3. Supply equipment and maintenance of sub centre
4. Record and reports
5. Training
6. MCH
7. Family welfare and MTP
8. Nutrition
9. Immunisation
10. Primary medical care
11. Health education.

Similarly social responsibilities of health worker female is described under the following heads:

1. MCH
2. FP
3. MTP
4. Nutrition
5. Communicable disease control
6. Traditional dai training
7. Collection of vital events
8. Record keeping
9. Primary health care
10. Other team activities for the community.

Social responsibilities for the health guide who is the member of the society itself is also described by the government and given as handout in the system by the Rural Health Division, Ministry of Health and FW, Government of India.

Home visiting and its extension to promote health of the public by discharging social responsibilities is made mandatory in Primary Health Care Services. Home help service is little wide area to provide the health care and social care services to the family to ensure sufficient support so that medial and social care in the home made practicable.

12

Social Trends and Social Issues

SOCIAL TRENDS

Trends are complex and overlapping which influence nursing education and nursing practice. Rapid development of knowledge, development of Science and Technology, excellent communication with the progress in the field of electronic technology are main trends that need consideration in nursing practice. A trend initially revolutionary will later become a standard at the national level in due course of time.

Table 12.1: Trends with related issues

Trends	Related issues
Knowledge expansion	Unlimited content Outdated textbooks Limited time Frequent change of curriculum Changed goals and expectations
Evidence based practice	Emphasis on only core element Depends on psychomotor skills Integration of best practice Different concepts Accreditation and regulations

cont..

cont..

Performance based learning	Class projects Collaboration Less lectures More learner responsibility Interactive learning strategy
Social, demographic, cultural, economic and political	More older people with geriatric problem Ethnic diversity, different custom Violence in civil life, Changed nurse-teacher relationship State and national policy on health care
Appropriate technology for community	Alternate health care Follow up of cases and active surveillance More planning Integration of work throughout Multiple agencies Rural based
Consumer orientation	Good alertness and attention Competent care Individual responsibility Shared responsibility and authority Balanced standards
Ethical concern	Ethical dilemmas Diverse beliefs Individual right of choice Incorporation in ordinance Accountability
Staff shortage	Limited clinical learning Heavy workload Fewer preceptors to help students Aging and retention results in issues for future of profession Problem of recruitment

cont..

cont..

More professional responsibilities	Validation of competence Preparedness for professional expectations High stress
Diversity, flexibility, mobility and delivery of education programmes	Internet courses Conflict of work and study Multiple entry for the course Multiple exit to course

SOCIAL ISSUES

Nursing education and nursing practice are influenced by umpteen number of related issues in our society. In previous chapter we have discussed at length number of major contemporary trends, which are due to different issues in the society. Any issue of the past can give rise to present trend and similarly any issue of today can give rise to future trend of the society. Thus Issue-Problem-Trend cycle is known as age old phenomenon.

Current social issues can be enumerated as under:

- Economics
- Finance
- Health care system
- Ethical
- Law
- Politics
- Social
- Culture
- Emergency care
- Information
- Indian systems of medicine
- Workplace.

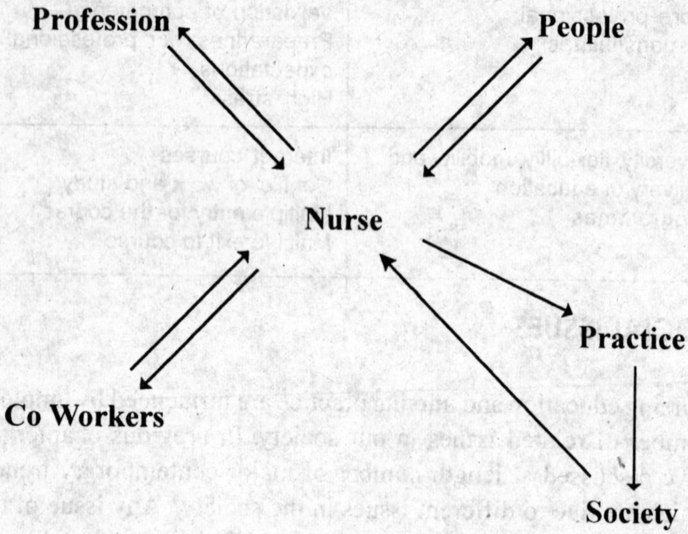

Fig.12.1: Interacting areas of social trends and social issues in nursing profession

13 Glossary of Sociology Words in Nursing

A

Absolute poverty	It is the lack of basic necessities like food, shelter and access to clean water and health care.
Accommodation	Mutual tolerance of ethnic group where the group live together peacefully with their distant identity
Active citizen	The citizen with prescribed duties and responsibilities for his society
Affluent society	High wages to many manual workers so that prosperity reached further down the class structure than ever before
Agrarian societies	Major form of employment in a society is agriculture
Ancient society	Greek and Roman society which was slave based production
Androcentric	Viewing the things from a male perspective
Anthropocentric	Viewing the human race in contrast to other species
Arranged marriage	Common in royal and aristocratic families where parents choose the marriage partner

B

Beanpole family	It is the result of one child families in the society
Behavior	Event of an individual which not intended or planned
Belief	Whatever we feel true and hold true

C

Capital	It is a social force in terms of money, machinery and plant to produce goods

Care in the community	It is a deinstitutionlisation policy for the care of sick and injured in their family and in their community
Case study	In-depth study of a group or an event
Caste	It is a system where social stratification is done in India
Citizenship	It defines the rights and responsibilities of individual by becoming a member of a nation or state
City	A large urban area with exciting and vibrant places
Civilisation	A complex cultural and social entity which covers a society
Culture clash	Is a cause of under achievement of working class and ethnic minority
Class culture	Is shared meanings and patterns of behavior associated with a particular social class
Classical sociologists	Early sociologists who developed distinctive way to look at society
Clinical sociology	An intervention to solve social problems in clinical practice
Closed society	Where little social mobility is seen
Cohabitation	Couple live together who are not legally married
Collective behavior	The action of mob or a crowd in a society
Community action	Community organised actions to achieve objectives in a locality
Compensatory education	Education which has as its main aim the overcoming of perceived deficiencies in a child's education
Compound family	Is a reconstituted family and is a feature of high divorce society which include step families
Comte	A French sociologist who developed the idea of positivism
Continuum	A social phenomenon showing variation between 2 opposite characteristics e.g., Hermaphrodite in between male and female
Contra culture	An alternative vision by a sub culture in a society
Core function of family	The sexual, the reproductive, the socialisation and the economic
Counter culture	Ideas, beliefs and practices of a sub culture
Cow sociology	Sociology of service of capitalist enterprises
Cross class family	Husband and wife in different social class by their occupation
Cross cultural comparison	Examination of two societies for similarities and differences
Crowd	Temporary and unorganized aggregation of human beings
Cultural taboos	Aspects of social life which are considered forbidden by the norms of society

Culture	Way of life of a society
Culture shock	Disruption because of an alien culture
Custom	Is an established pattern and a traditional pattern of human behavior

D

Death of the family	Family weaning by divorce, cohabitation and lone parent
Delinquency	Antisocial actions
Democratic socialism	Socialist society is got by an electoral process
Density	Describes urbanism
Dependency ratio	Describes young and old dependents on head of family
Development	Process where society moves to an industrial state
Dharma	A belief in Hinduism
Division of labour	Part of activities done for survival and sustenance where specialisation exists
Divorce	The legal termination of a marriage
Diversity	Can be cultural diversity or diversity in nursing education programme
Downward social mobility	Poor health and tough business allow a super ordinate to move downward
Durkheim	French sociologist who developed functionalism

E

Egoism	It is a cult of the individual
Emotions	Feelings like love, hate
Empty nest family	Children moved out of adult partners
Ethos	Particular social and cultural characteristics and norms of a group

F

Family	People related to by blood and marriage live
Family size	Number of children born to a couple
Family structure	The composition of a group of people living together as family
Feudal society	Depending on possession or non possession of land, people are ordered in a strict hierarchy
Folk society	Rural societies in which everyone knows everyone else
Folkways	The recognized or accepted ways of behaving in society

G

Giddens	British sociologist who developed structuration theory
Global village	An idea of mass communication by film and TV

H

Health	Problematic nature of concepts of both health and disease "not merely the absence of disease and infirmity, but complete physical, mental and social well-being"
Hegemony	Simultaneous consent by masses to the type of society imposed upon them by the dominant group in society
Hierarchy of needs	This is Maslow theory which describes physiological needs such as food and shelter, safety and security, love, companionship and affection, self esteem and the esteem of others, self actualization (i.e., realising one's potential to the fullest)
High culture	Opera, ballet, sculpture and such arts patronised by elite in society, to reach different audience
Household	Individual or group have same address and share meal and living accommodation
Hydraulic society	Survival depend on appropriate irrigation where ancient culture depended on access to water

I

I Q	It is a measure of a person's intelligence by a test
Icons	Signs and pictures representing some meaning in a society e.g.., Om = Hindu, Moon = Muslim, Cross = Christian etc.,
Indicators of class	Both by objective and subjective an individual's exact class position is ascertained

J

Juvenile delinquency	Disorder and disruption caused by young in a society

L

Laws	Codified mores
Leisure society	Is a predicted automation which help to enjoy leisure activities as their central life interest

M

Macro sociology	Large scale focus on a society with functionalism
Marx	A classical sociologist. His followers seized power. Industrial sociology and class analysis emphasised
Mass culture	Modern leisure is often provided for people in large number
Mass society	Society where individual are atomised attached to hardly any group between power and the group
Mores	Group routines necessary for continued existence.

N

Neo Marxism	Updating the insights of Marx by a group
New social movement	(NSM) Interests and identities such as gender, ethnicity, sexuality, religious feeling etc.,
Norms	Social rules which define what is expected of individuals in certain situations
Nuclear family	Consists adult male, adult female and children

O

Over urbanisation	The conditions of insecurity which affect many of the inhabitants of cities in the third world

P

Pedagogy	The science of teaching
Political socialisation	Individuals are initiated into the dominant values and traditions of a society
Popular culture	The mass features of the media in post modern societies
Poverty cycle	Explanation of how poverty is transmitted from generation to generation

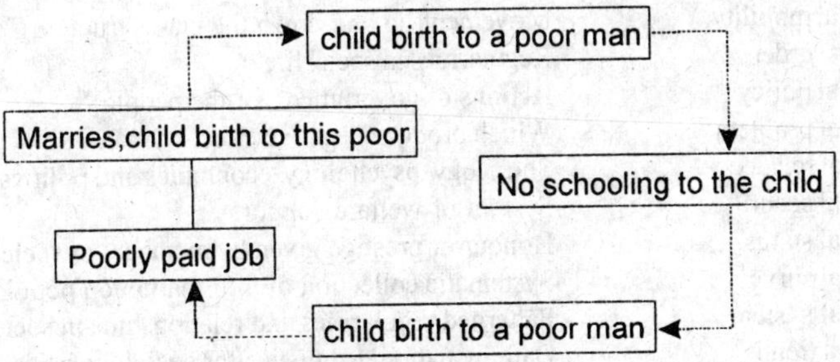

Figure 13.1: Poverty cycle

Pygmalion effect	Way in which expectations and consistent behavior by social actors can shape the behavior of others in society
Pygmalion effect	Way in which expectations and consistent behavior by social actors can shape the behavior of others in society

R

Reconstituted family	Children living with step parents, step brothers and step sisters
Relative poverty	State of being poor with reference to a real or perceived standard of living in a society
Remarriage	Divorced individual enters a marriage contract for a second time or more times
Risk society	Modern world with sense of danger and challenges
Role	The expected pattern of behavior associated with a social status
ROSLA (rising of school leaving age)	Accepted normal programmes of study and examina tions to allow to leave school early

S

Semiotics	Signs in society for media and myths
Social action	Direct or indirect interaction
Social benefit	Financial benefit through states
Social change	Aspects of society move from one state to another
Social class	Hierarchical divisions of society by wealth, income and occupation
Social closure	Monopoly of privileges and rewards for themselves
Social construction	Built up phenomenon by social process
Social consumption	Use of goods and services
Social contract	Utilitarian agreement in society
Social control	Social conformity to the dominant values and norms
Social engineering	Social change by social policy
Social mobility	Movement up and down the class structure
Social order	Regularities in social life
Social policy	Actions of government for the people
Social problem	Which produce negative effect on man
Social science	Sociology, psychology, economics and politics
Social security	System of welfare support
Social status	Honour or prestige given by members of society
Social survey	Systematic collection of information on population
Social system	Patterned regularities and relationships in society
Social trend	Data by national statistics for sociologists

Socialization	Learning values, ideas, practices and roles of society
Society	The social totality of all the relationships in a given space
Sociobiology	Approach to human conduct by biological imperatives
Sociometry	Moreno method for information on how the members feel about each other
Styles of life	Goods that people consume and taste that they exhibit
Sub culture	Society group sharing common values
Subjective poverty	Feels poor by comparisons
Sub urbanisation	City develop outlying districts
Suburbia	City area where majority live
Super class	Fat cats like director of firm, lawyer, investment manager

T

Taboo	That which is forbidden by religious law or by custom
30:30:40 Society	Advantaged 40%, a newly insecure 30% and a disadvantaged 30% in a society
Tradition	Transmission of body of laws from generation to generation
Three roads to modernity	Capitalism, state socialism and state capitalism

U

Underclass	People at bottom of class system
Undeveloped society	Original state of a society with no development
Unemployment	Working age people but without work
Upward social mobility	Movement from a subordinate social position to a higher one
Urban apartheid	Segregate space in a class specific way like private space for rich, ghettos for the poor
Urban areas	High population density area
Urban crisis	Modern class struggle, unmet welfare
Urban social movement	Collective interest in community with concern
Urban villager	Working class in city
Urban zone	Urban process in spread out zones

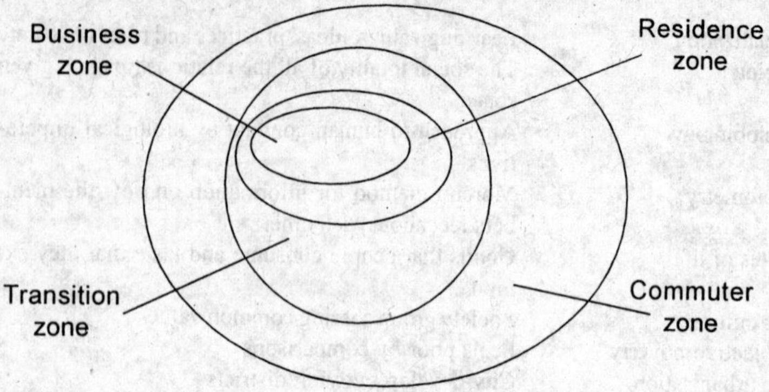

Figure 13.2: Urban zones

V

Values	Ideas and beliefs, which are thought to be valuable

W

Weber	Classical sociologists gave ideas of social change

Y

Youth culture	Way of life and attitude same in youths

Appendix

(Nursing Council of India Syllabus)

SOCIOLOGY

Introduction

Definition of sociology, Nature and scope of the discipline, importance and application of sociology in nursing.

Individual & society

Society and community, Nature of society, Difference between society and community, Process of socialisation and individualisation, Personal disorganisation.

Culture

Nature of culture, Evolution of culture, Diversity and uniformity of culture, Culture and socialisation, Trans-cultural society, Influence on health and disease.

Social groups and processes

The meaning and classification of groups, Primary and secondary group, In group v/s out-group, class tribe, caste, Economic, political, religious groups, mob, crowd, public and audience interaction and social processes, Cooperation, competition, conflict, Accommodation, assimilation and isolation.

Population

Society and population, Population distribution in India, demographic characteristics, Malthusian theory of population, Population explosion in India and its impact on health status, Family welfare programmes.

Family and marriage

Family — functions, Types, joint, nuclear, blended and extended family characteristics, the modern family- changes, problems, dowry etc welfare services, Changes and legislations on family and marriage in India -marriage Acts; Marriage — forms and functions of marriage, marriage and family problems in India, Family, marriage and their influence on health and health practices.

Social stratification

Meaning and types of social stratification, The Indian Caste system–origin and features, Features of caste in India today, Social class system and status, social mobility- meaning and types, Race as a biological concept, criteria of racial classification, salient features of primary races, racism — Influence of class, caste and race on health and health practices.

Types of communities in India (Rural, Urban & Regional)

Features of village community & characteristics of Indian villages Panchayat system, social dynamics, Community development project and planning, Changes in Indian rural life, Availability of health facilities in rural and its impact on health and health practices; Urban- community- features. The grown cities, urbanisation and its impact on health and health practices, major urban problems- urban slums; Region — problems and impact on health.

Social change

Nature and process of social change, Factors influencing social change — cultural change, cultural lag; Introduction to theories of social change — linear, cyclical, Marxian, functional, Role of nurse-change agents.

Social organisation and social system

Social organisation — elements, types; Democratic and authoritarian modes of participation, Voluntary associations: Social system — role and status as structural elements of social system, Inter-relationships of institutions.

Social control

Nature and process of social control, Political, legal, religious, educational, economic, industrial and technological systems; norms and values - folkways and more, customs, laws and fashion; role of nurse.

Social problems

Social disorganisation, Control & planning ; poverty, housing, illiteracy, food supplies, prostitution, rights of women and children, vulnerable groups; elderly, handicapped, minority groups and other marginalised groups, child labour, child abuse, delinquency and crime, substance abuse, HIV/AIDS, social welfare programmes in India; Role of nurse.

PSYCHOLOGY

Introduction

History and origin of science of psychology, Definitions and scope of psychology, Relevance to nursing, Methods of psychology.

Biology of behaviour

Body mind relationship modulation process in health and illness, Genetics and behaviour, heredity and environment — Brain and behaviour; nervous system, neurons and synapse, Association cortex, right and left hemispheres, Psychology of sensations, Muscular and glandular controls of behaviour of an organism/integrated responses.

Cognitive process

Attention — types determinants duration & degree alterations, Perception meaning principles factors affecting errors, Learning nature types learner and learning factors influencing laws and theories process transfer study habits; Memory — meaning, types, nature, factors influencing, development theories and methods of memorising and forgetting, thinking — types and levels, stages of development, relationship with language and communication; Intelligence — meaning, classification, uses, theories: Aptitude — concept, types, individual differences and variability, Psychometric assessments of cognitive process, Alterations in cognitive process, Applications.

Motivation and emotional process

Motivation — meaning, concepts, types, theories, motives and behaviour, conflicts and frustration, conflict resolution; emotion and stress — emotion, definition, components, changes in emotions, theories, emotional adjustments, emotions in health and illness; Stress — stressors, cycle, effect, adaptation and coping; Attitude — meaning, nature, development, factors affecting; Behaviour and attitudes, Attitudinal change, Psychometric assessments of emotions and attitudes, Alterations in emotions, applications.

Personality

Definitions, topography, types, theories, Psychometric assessments of personality, Alterations in personality, Applications.

Developmental psychology

Psychology of people at different ages from infancy to old age, Psychology of vulnerable individuals – challenged, women, sick etc., Psychology of groups.

Mental hygiene and mental health

Concepts of mental hygiene and mental health, characteristics of mentally healthy person, Warning signs of poor mental health, Promotive and preventive mental health strategies and services, Ego defence mechanisms and implications, Personal and social adjustments, Guidance and counselling, Role of nurse.

Psychological assessment and tests

Types development, characteristics, Principle, uses, interpretations and role of nurse in psychological assessment.

PSYCHIATRY

Introduction

Mental health, abnormal behaviour.

Defence mechanism of human body

Ego defence mechanisms, repression, sublimation, reaction formation, dissociation, conversion, rationalisation, projection, regression.

Common mental disorders classified

Schizophrenia, Maniac depressive psychosis, Paranoia.

Therapeutic nurse patient relationships

Psychoanalytic model, Behavioural model

Psychosomatic disorders

Causes, management.

Individual in society with chrematistic disorders

Sexual disorders, Substance dependence, sociopath reaction, Childhood disorders.

Modern therapy in Psychiatry

Crisis situation

Community Psychiatry

Primary, secondary and tertiary prevention.

ANTHROPOLOGY

Introduction

Physical, Cultural, social.

Ethnology

Totemism – custom associated activities

SOCIAL SCIENCES

Psychology, Child Psychology, Adult and old age psychology

Sociology

Family, individual, joint, culture, social problems, social and community problems, laws,

Economics

National income, social security, Population explosion, family budgeting, Industrialisation.

INDEX